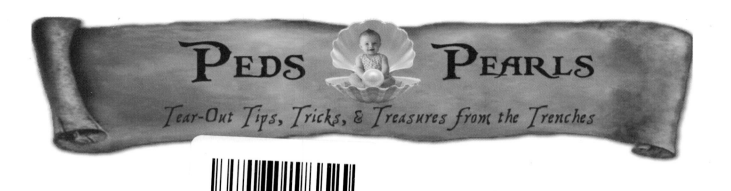

PEDS PEARLS

Tear-Out Tips, Tricks, & Treasures from the Trenches

Scott L. DeBoer RN, MSN, CPEN, CEN, CCRN, CFRN, EMT-P

Founder

Pedi-Ed-Trics Emergency Medical Solutions

Critical Care Transport/Emergency Nurse

Editors and Clinical Advisers

Julie L. Bacon MSN-HCSM, RNC-LRN, NE-BC, CPN, CPEN, C-NPT

Emily C. Dawson MD

Michael Seaver RN, BA

"You make 'em, I amuse 'em"

Dr. Seuss

Printed in the United States of America

ISBN 978-0-692-61269-9

© 2016 - Pedi-Ed-Trics Emergency Medical Solutions, LLC

This review book is designed to provide accurate information in regard to the subject matter. The handbook and its recommendations are based upon the author's review of current nursing and medical research and do not represent the policies of the author's or editors' places of employment. In publishing this book, neither the author, nor the editors or publisher are engaged in rendering nursing, medical, or other professional services. If nursing, medical, or other expert assistance is required, the services of a competent professional should be sought.

*Purchase additional copies of Peds Pearls at www.PediEd.com

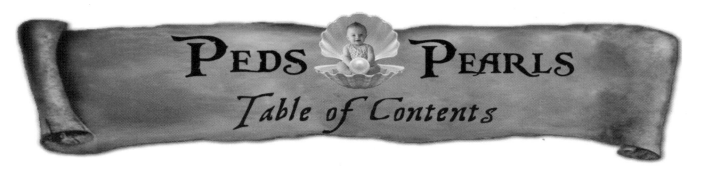

Table of Contents

1 - 5, 5, and 15 ~ *Simple Febrile Seizures*

2 - When in Doubt...Sit 'Em Out ~ *Pediatric Concussions*

3 - Adult Vs. Pediatric ABCs ~ *Beyond Airway, Breathing, and Circulation*

4 - Asthma ABCs : Airways Being Constricted ~ *Bagging Asthmatics*

5 - B5: Big Blue Blotches That Don't Blanch...Bad! ~ *Meningococcemia*

6 - Bad Bellies ~ *Crucial Clues and Abdominal Assessments*

7 - Barking, Boogers, Steeples, and Steroids ~ *Croup*

8 - Big Head, Little Body Syndrome ~ *Implications for Medical and Trauma Care*

9 - Big Parts and Little Parts ~ *Burns and the Rule of 9s*

10 - Bigger Vs. Better Vs. Nothing? ~ *Choosing Bag and Mask Sizes*

11 - Catch, Clean, and Clamp ~ *Emergency Newborn Care*

12 - Consultations, Custody, and Crashing Children ~ *Emergency Protective Custody*

13 - Crashing Kids with Congenital Cardiac Conditions ~ *Congenital Heart Disease*

14 - Cuffed Tubes in Kids...Crazy or Correct? ~ *Uncuffed Vs. Cuffed Endotracheal Tubes*

15 - Dead, Dead, Dead, and Dead ~ *Emergency Burn Care*

16 - Fast, Furious, Drooling, and Dying ~ *Epiglottitis*

17 - Five Tiny Trauma Triads ~ *Bad Things Come in Threes*

18 - Goobers, Glucose, Snot, and Sugar ~ *CSF Leaks*

19 - Guns, Drills, Bones, and Babies ~ *Intraosseous Access: The Basics*

20 - Guns, Drills, Bones, and Babies ~ *Intraosseous Access: Beyond the Basics*

21 - Keep 'Em Pink, Warm, and Sweet...Everything Else is Fluff ~ *Pre-Transport Pediatric Priorities*

22 - Killer Kuffs Vs. Cute Children ~ *Look at the Child, Not Only the Numbers*

23 - When Thunder Roars, Go Indoors! ~ *Lightning Injuries*

24 - Allegations and Algebra? ~ *Medication Malpractice*

25 - Doses and Decimals ~ *Medical Malpractice*

26 - Perils of Potassium ~ *Medical Malpractice*

27 - Mg and mL... Moving and Pushing... ~ *Administering Epinephrine and Amiodarone*

28 - Misadventures in Airway Management ~ *Verification of Endotracheal Tube Placement*

29 - Nebs 101 - Closer is Better ~ *Pediatric Nebulizer Techniques*

30 - Not Dead...Only Half Dead ~ *Pediatric Cardioversion*

31 - Only Two Kinds of Brains... Happy & Unhappy ~ *Neuropathology Made Easy*

32 - Passing TNCC and ENPC ~ *Top Ten Test Taking Tips*

33 - Pediatric Defibrillation ~ *Easy as 1, 2, or More! - Pediatric Defibrillation Tips*

34 - Pediatric Parkland ~ *Fluid Resuscitation and Burns*

35 - Prayer and Parents Vs. Diabetes and Death ~ *Religious Objections and Emergency Medical Care*

36 - Rabies: Reality and the Urban Legends ~ *Emergency Prevention and Management of Rabies*

37 - Raccoons, Battles, and Drums ~ *Basilar Skull Fractures*

38 - Sandbags, Suffering, Epidurals, and Every Breath You Take ~ *Flail Chests*

39 - Scared of Shunts? ~ *Assessment and Management of Sick Shunts*

40 - Shaken, Not Stirred ~ *Shaken Baby Syndrome*

41 - Suffering, Suffocating, and Stroking ~ *Sickle Cell Emergencies*

42 - Fighting the Fangs ~ *Snake Bite Basics, Do's and Don'ts*

43 - Something Doesn't Fit ~ *DKA Vs. Drugs*

44 - Negotiating with Kidnappers? ~ *Special Needs Children*

45 - TET Terrors ~ *Tetralogy of Fallot*

46 - Stop, Drop, and Squat (or Sedate) ~ *Tetralogy of Fallot and TET Spells*

47 - Bearing, Blowing, and Bags ~ *Emergency Management of Pediatric SVT*

48 - Call 911 or Go to the Closest ER ~ *Telephone Triage and Medical Malpractice*

49 - The "B's" of Abuse ~ *Non-Accidental Trauma and Child Abuse*

50 - Torsions and Twisted Testicles ~ *Testicular Torsion*

51 - Volvulus Begins with V ~ *Assessment and Management of Pediatric Volvulus*

52 - What Size, How Much, and Where... Every Kid, Every Time ~ *Airways, Epinephrine, and Intraosseous*

✦ *Bonus Christmas Pearl*

53- Christmas Carols and Critical Communications ~ *"Do You Hear What I Hear?"*

If you and your staff are enjoying these Peds Pearls, help spread the word!

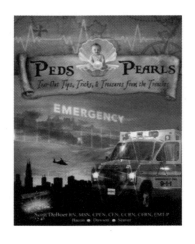

PEDS PEARLS

About the Author

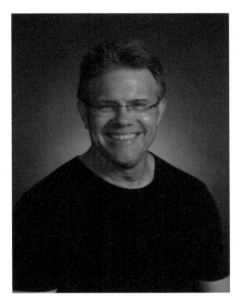

Scott DeBoer RN, MSN, CEN, CCRN, CFRN, CPEN, EMT-P, is an internationally recognized pediatric emergency nurse expert, author of six pediatric emergency related books, and co-author of over 100 medical articles for nurses, paramedics, and respiratory therapists. In addition to his extensive training in emergency, critical care, and flight nursing, Scott is the primary seminar leader for Pedi-Ed-Trics Emergency Medical Solutions, a seminar company he founded and dedicated to saving the lives of children through education. He has been presenting to thousands of medical professionals around the world for over 20 years.

Scott retired from the University of Chicago Aeromedical Network (UCAN) in 2015 where he worked for over 20 years as a flight nurse. Scott also worked as a neonatal, pediatric & adult flight nurse for Life Flight in Peoria, IL as well as being a part of the flight and rescue team in the Grand Canyon for Classic Lifeguard. Scott has held staff nurse positions in intensive care and emergency/trauma nursing for over 25 years. He also spent some time as a clinical nursing instructor at Purdue University and is a current member of AACN, ENA, and ASTNA. In addition, Scott serves as a legal nurse consultant with various national law firms as an expert witness for nursing and EMS malpractice issues.

In 1994 Scott married Lisa Banter-DeBoer and they have two teenage children. Scott and Lisa have owned and operated Pedi-Ed-Trics (formerly Peds-R-Us) together since the late 1990's. Even with nearly 50 teaching engagements on neonatal, pediatric, & "big-people" emergency topics somewhere in the world every year, Scott still manages to find time to homeschool his daughter, coordinate events at his church, and hold certifications in emergency, critical care, trauma, and flight nursing.

ACKNOWLEDGEMENTS

Lisa DeBoer... President of Pedi-Ed-Trics Emergency Medical Solutions and my wife of over 20 years. It has been amazing to see your paramedic to pediatric president speaking career continue to blossom, as well as your love of all things cardiac incorporated into our pediatric skills labs as they continue to evolve into what you envisioned so many years ago. Thank you for continuing to be an inspiration and blessing to me, our children, and so many others.

Joshua DeBoer, age 19, and **Nina DeBoer**, age 17... Thank you for all of your stat computer services and emergency late-night pastry preparations. I couldn't have completed this first round of Peds Pearls without you!

Gabriella Baez... aka. hip and trendy girl, the director of all things marketing and social media, as well as the newest member of the Pedi-Ed-Trics family. Lisa and I are so glad you decided to come play with us.

PEDS PEARLS
Editors & Clinical Advisers

Editor: Michael Seaver RN, BA

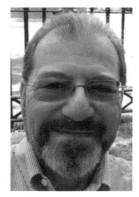

Michael Seaver is an experienced pre-hospital provider, nurse, informaticist, and is an internationally recognized conference presenter, author, and editor. He has served on the EMS Commission for the state of Indiana, and has been an instructor for PHTLS, TNCC, ENPC, ACLS, PALS, and NRP courses. He is a life member of the Emergency Nurses Association and has served as the Emergency Department Technology Special Interest Group facilitator and chaired the ENA's Technology and Informatics Workgroup. He currently provides clinical and technology consulting services to healthcare organizations. Michael also acts as an expert consultant on medical-legal cases involving technology and electronic documentation issues.

Editorial and Clinical Adviser: Julie L. Bacon, MSN-HCSM, RNC-LRN, NE-BC, CPN, CPEN, C-NPT

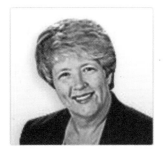

Julie Bacon is the Chief Flight Nurse and Manager of the Patient Transfer Center at All Children's Hospital in St. Petersburg, Florida. Passionate about pediatric and neonatal education, she is a frequent speaker at conferences and hospitals nationwide. She has served as the Florida EMS for Children Advisory Committee Chair since 2007.

Editorial and Clinical Adviser: Emily C. Dawson MD

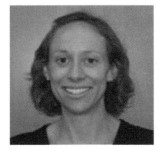

Emily Dawson is a triple boarded physician in Pediatrics, Pediatric Emergency Medicine and Pediatric Critical Care. She is also the director of the pediatric sepsis initiative at Comer Children's Hospital in Chicago, Illinois. She takes an active role as an educator for pediatric nurses, residents and fellows as well as medical students.

Pedi-Ed-Trics™

Emergency Medical Solutions, LLC

Education... The Heart Of All We Do

A NOTE FROM SCOTT:

I'd like to especially thank all of my editors, clinical advisers and contributors to this, our first Peds Pearls book. Your tireless contributions to this project were invaluable and I cannot thank all of you enough. If it were not for all of your countless hours of work and devotion to the importance of pediatric emergency care, this book would never have been possible. It is with the utmost respect and appreciation that I would personally like to thank each of you for sharing your expertise.

Scott

Scott DeBoer RN, MSN, CPEN, CEN, CCRN, CFRN, EMT-P
Author, Pedi-Ed-Trics Founder, Your Friend

P.S. If you are a pediatric expert (nurse, medic, doc, or RT) or have a great peds tip you would like to share with other medical professionals, please email me your idea for possible inclusion in our future editions of Peds Pearls: Tips and Tricks from the Trenches. Feel free to email me directly: Scott@PediEd.com.

1-888-280-PEDS (7337)

9052 Beall Street, Suite B, Dyer, IN 46311 • Fax: 1-866-449-PEDS (7337) • Info@PediEd.com • PediEd.com

PEDS PEARLS
Contributors

Peter Antevy MD
    Founder and Chief Medical Officer
    Pediatric Emergency Standards, Inc.
    Davie, Florida

Gabriella Baez
    Director of Marketing and Social Media
    Pedi-Ed-Trics Emergency Medical Solutions, LLC
    Dyer, Indiana

Marlene L. Bokholdt MS, RN, CPEN
    Senior Associate
    Institute for Emergency Nursing
    Emergency Nurses Association
    Des Plaines, Illinois

Maria Broadstreet RN, MSN, CPNP
    Pediatric Nurse Practitioner
    Department of Pediatric Cardiovascular Surgery
    Lurie Children's Hospital
    Chicago, Illinois

James Broselow MD
    Creator: Broselow Tape
    Medical Director: eBroselow, LLC
    Raleigh, North Carolina

Teri Campbell RN, BSN, CEN, CFRN
    Flight Nurse: UCAN
    University of Chicago Medicine
    Chicago, Illinois

John R. Clark JD, MBA, NRP, FP-C, CCP-C, CMTE
Chief Operating Officer
International Board of Specialty Certification
Carmel, Indiana

Lisa DeBoer
President
Pedi-Ed-Trics Emergency Medical Solutions, LLC
Dyer, Indiana

Vickie Dollhausen, RN, MSN, CEN, CPEN, EMT-P
Clinical Nurse Educator
Sacred Heart Health System
Pensacola, Florida

J. Robert Gbur MT (ASCP)
Medical Technologist
Franciscan Health Rensselaer
Rensselaer, Indiana

Daniel Griffin AS, CCEMT-P
EMS Educator
DJ Griffin Education, LLC
Gainesville, Florida

Joie Hickenbottom RN, EMT-P, CEN
Pediatric Transport Nurse
American Family Children's Hospital: CHETA
Flight Nurse: UW Med Flight
Madison, Wisconsin

Judith Holleman MSN, RN, CCRN, PCPNP-BC, PNP-AC
Pediatric Nurse Practitioner
Section of Pediatric Neurosurgery
Comer Children's Hospital
University of Chicago Medicine
Chicago, Illinois

Michael R. Lovelace, RN, CEN, CFRN, CTRN, TCRN, CCEMTP, NREMTP, EMTP-T
UAB School of Medicine
Department of Emergency Medicine
EMS Program Coordinator
Birmingham, Alabama

Bonnie Lundblom RN, BSN, CPEN
Nurse Consultant: eBroselow (1998-2014)
Jacksonville, Florida

Stu McVicar RRT, FP-C, CCEMT-P
Pediatric Transport Respiratory Therapist
American Family Children's Hospital: CHETA
UW Med Flight
Madison, Wisconsin

Justin Milici, MSN, RN, CEN, CPEN, CFRN, CCRN, FAEN
Clinical Educator: Emergency Services
Parkland Health and Hospital System
Dallas, Texas

Suzanne Mindlin
Attorney-at-Law focusing on medical malpractice
San Diego, California

Annemarie O'Connor MSN, FNP-BC, APN/CNP
Nurse Practitioner: Burn Center
University of Chicago Medicine
Chicago, Illinois

Leigh Ann Pansch, MSN, FNP-BC
Advanced Practice Nurse
Dermatologists of Southwest Ohio
Cincinnati, Ohio

Jacci Patterson RN, BSN
> Vice President of Clinical Content
> eBroselow, LLC
> Raleigh, North Carolina

Steven Rogge RN, CEN, CCRN, CFRN, FAWM
> Flight Nurse: Airlift Northwest
> Staff Nurse: Neonatal ICU
> University of Washington Medical Center
> Seattle, Washington

Michael Rushing CCEMT-P, RN, NRP, BSN, CEN, CPEN, CFRN, CCRN-CMC
> Flight Nurse: Lifeguard 1
> Lifeguard Santa Rosa County
> Milton, Florida

Rebecca Sosa
> Artist and Illustrator
> Saint John, Indiana

Christopher Speaker RN, MSN, APN, FNP-BC, CPN
> Nurse Practitioner
> Department of Pediatric Surgery
> Comer Children's Hospital
> University of Chicago Medicine
> Chicago, Illinois

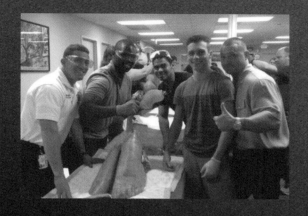
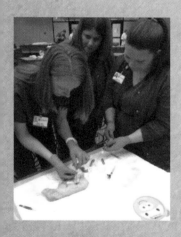
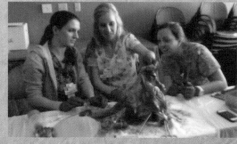

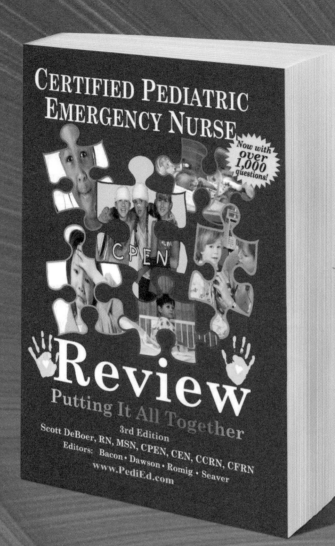
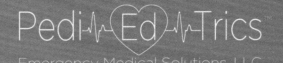

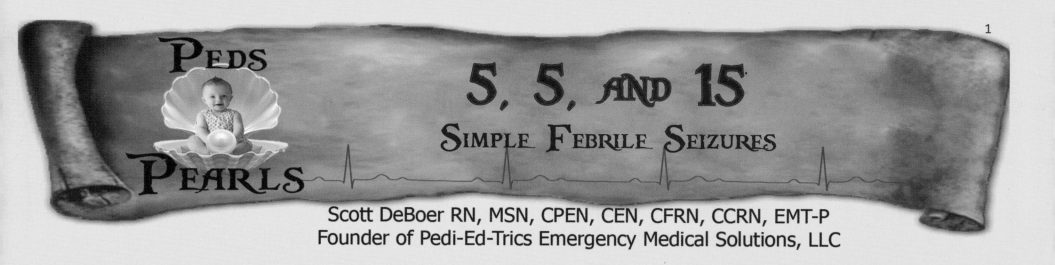

5, 5, AND 15
SIMPLE FEBRILE SEIZURES

Scott DeBoer RN, MSN, CPEN, CEN, CFRN, CCRN, EMT-P
Founder of Pedi-Ed-Trics Emergency Medical Solutions, LLC

Parents, especially new, first time parents, go through lots of scary events. For many, one of the scariest is when their little one has a fever. And even scarier than a fever, is when a seizure piggy backs on that fever. That's what we, in the medical field, call a febrile seizure. Quite simply, it is when a child has a seizure brought on by a fever.

For most of us, seasoned medical professionals that we are, a febrile seizure does not evoke the same frightened concern that a new parent might experience. Our cool, calm, and collected approach to these patients and parents should be the result of our differentiating the febrile seizure from any other, more serious type of seizure activity in children.

So, when it comes to recognizing the pediatric febrile seizure, just remember three things. And the key to jog your memory is **5, 5, & 15**! (Notice how "febrile seizure" starts with "f" and our memory key is three words that start with "f"s!)

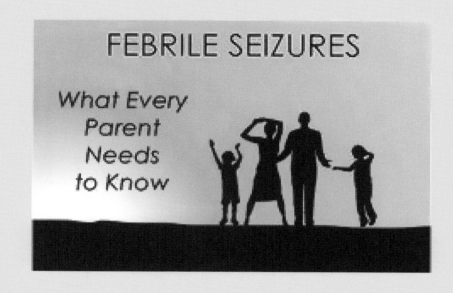

So, as healthcare providers, what we need to remember about this most common type of pediatric seizure is **5, 5, & 15**. But what about parents? We need to treat them, as well as their children. They need to have two basic questions addressed prior to leaving the ER, because we know that the parents are worried about these things.

Question #1 - *Does the fact that the child had a simple febrile seizure mean that s/he has or is going to develop epilepsy?* Absolutely not. One has little to nothing to do with the other. Having a febrile seizure DOES NOT mean the child will develop epilepsy. The vast majority of kids experiencing a febrile seizure (upwards of 95%) do not have any further complications from the seizure.

Question #2 *Will it happen again?* Very possibly. Up to 1/3 of kids who have a febrile seizure will have another one (or two) before they outgrow them… and there's typically nothing we can do to prevent them. Anticonvulsants (phenobarbital, etc.) or prophylactic fever prevention with Tylenol (acetaminophen) or Motrin (ibuprofen) have **not** been shown to have an effect on the likelihood of having another febrile seizure.

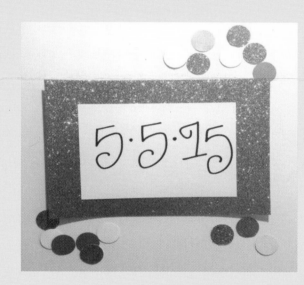

(F)ive- The little one is under the age of **5**. Febrile seizures are especially common in toddlers when a fever, added to the normal brain development, causes chaos! (The caveat here is the knowledge that infants under the age of six-months are the exception to this recognition rule. Seizures in kids younger than 6-months-old tend to be something other than febrile in nature.)

(F)ive- The kids with febrile seizures typically have temperatures in the 102-10**5**°F (38.9-40.5°C) range. It's not necessarily the highest point of the fever, but in many cases, is a result of how fast the fever rises.

(F)ifteen- The seizure lasts for less than **15** minutes. Seizures lasting longer than 15 minutes are probably something besides a **simple** febrile seizure.

If the child has a second febrile seizure, the child should certainly be brought in for evaluation. But it is important to remember that the second (or subsequent) febrile seizure is not an unexpected occurrence. The parents are still going to be concerned and this is certainly understandable. But a little preparation really does go a long way. So, before the kid goes home after a first simple febrile seizure, make sure to address those two crucial questions with the caregivers. Healthcare professionals… we just need to remember **5, 5, and 15**!

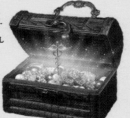

Info@PediEd.com ☏ 1-888-280-PEDS (7337) ☏ PediEd.com

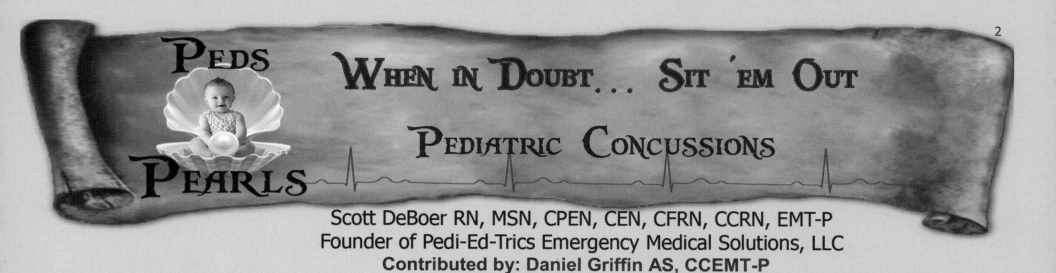

When in Doubt... Sit 'em Out

Pediatric Concussions

Scott DeBoer RN, MSN, CPEN, CEN, CFRN, CCRN, EMT-P
Founder of Pedi-Ed-Trics Emergency Medical Solutions, LLC
Contributed by: Daniel Griffin AS, CCEMT-P

Kids love to play. As they get older, involvement in organized sporting activities is a common step in their growth and development. Participation in sporting activities, at all levels, provides much needed exercise and socialization as well as physical and mental challenges. But unfortunately, these activities also provide many opportunities for injuries. One type of injury, particularly common in contact sports, is the concussion. A concussion is a form of mild traumatic brain injury (MTBI) that affects the brain's cognitive and physical functions; it is caused by a direct or indirect blow to the head or upper torso.

The evaluation for a possible concussion should include both physical and cognitive assessment elements and is the KEY to determining whether or not the player should be removed from the game. Common practice used to be to merely "shake it off" when a possible concussion was sustained, but current best practice is simply, "When in doubt, sit them out." A comprehensive evaluation should be conducted in an Emergency Department or a physician's office and should focus on both physical and cognitive symptoms. Additionally, any sleep or emotional changes that might occur should be identified and noted.

Physical Assessment: In addition to your normal assessments for head injuries, specific steps to look for a possible concussion include:

- Level of consciousness changes
- Neck pain
- Balance problems
- Dizziness
- Visual disturbances
- Hearing and/or light sensitivity
- Headaches
- Unstable or unsteady gait

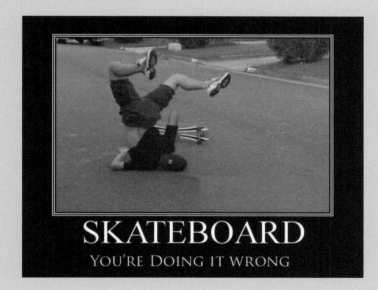

SKATEBOARD
YOU'RE DOING IT WRONG

It is important to note that a loss of consciousness occurs in <u>less than 10%</u> of concussed patients and is <u>not</u> an indication of concussion severity. Concussions cannot be diagnosed through the use of X-rays, CT scans, or MRIs since they are functional, not structural injuries.

From the Acute Concussion Evaluation (ACE) checklist: www.cdc.gov

Cognitive Assessment: Ask questions to test memory and cognitive functions such as:

- How do you feel?
- What team were you playing against?
- Who scored last?
- What day of the week is it?
- What month is it?
- Can you name the months of the year in reverse order? (if age appropriate)

Sleep Assessment: Is the person drowsy? Is she sleeping more (or less) than normal? Is he having difficulty falling asleep?

Emotional Assessment: Be alert for emotional changes. Is he more irritable or nervous than usual? Do you notice unexpected sadness or giddiness? Is she more emotional than normal?

Treatment: In the pre-hospital setting, treat possible concussions according to local EMS protocols. After a physician evaluation, commonly recommended treatment involves cognitive rest including <u>no</u> homework (they will love this part), but also <u>no</u> video games, TV, cell phone usage, computers, or sports activities (they are not so thrilled with this part) until symptoms have fully resolved. As the patient remains symptom free, we would expect a gradually increasing program of physical activities under the guidance of a qualified athletic trainer or physician.

Equipment Concerns: Visit your local schools to identify the types of protective sports equipment that are used and what steps are necessary to remove that equipment (especially for airway access and spinal cord precautions). It is not uncommon for schools and community programs to have multiple types of equipment with different methods of removal.

All 50 states have concussion laws in place. Most laws require that the patient be evaluated by a physician trained in sports medicine/concussion management before returning to play. The patients should be told to expect they will not be returning to the activity anytime soon (especially during the same game or practice session). There is absolutely no return to play on the same day!

Symptoms <u>usually</u> resolve within 7-10 days. However, patients with more severe concussions or with a history of previous concussions may remain symptomatic for many months. Additionally, younger children's brains are still developing and often take longer to recover from a concussion.

Final Thoughts

An injury which might produce a concussion should never be referred to as "getting your bell rung" or "just a ding, so walk it off." Concussions are mild TRAUMAtic brain injuries and we must take them seriously.

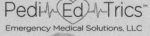

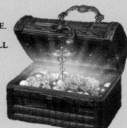

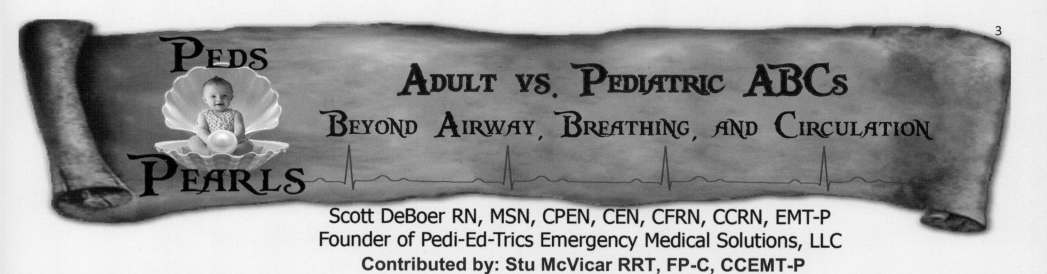

Peds Pearls

Adult vs. Pediatric ABCs
Beyond Airway, Breathing, and Circulation

Scott DeBoer RN, MSN, CPEN, CEN, CFRN, CCRN, EMT-P
Founder of Pedi-Ed-Trics Emergency Medical Solutions, LLC
Contributed by: Stu McVicar RRT, FP-C, CCEMT-P

"ABCDEFG… Now I know my ABCs…" This song has been drilled into our heads since, well, since as long as we can remember! And it didn't end when we started school. We still have to know our ABCs throughout our healthcare careers. Early on while working as a flight medic/RT, I learned to break down the ABCs into adult and pediatric versions.

ABC

Adult ABCs stands for ALWAYS BRING CAMERA! If you have had the experience of flying in a helicopter on the night of a Chicago Cubs game at Wrigley Field, a Green Bay Packers game at Lambeau Field, or even better, a Grateful Dead concert in Las Vegas, it is very likely that before the evening is over, you will have seen some of the most bizarre things in your career.

> *Legal/Risk Management Note:*
> *Healthcare regulations tend to disagree with the camera concept and suggest, rather strongly, that you stay with the Airway, Breathing, Circulation version learned in CPR class.*

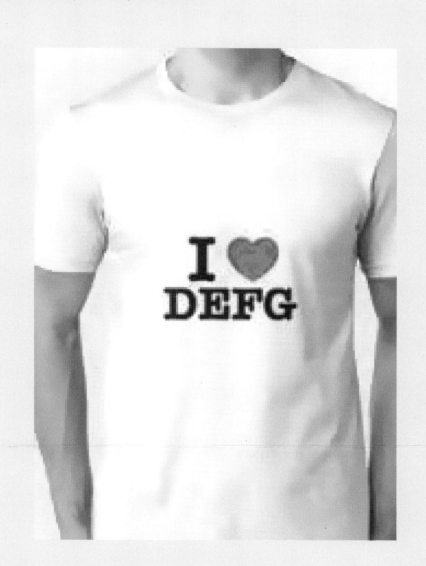

Pediatric ABCs are a bit different. ABC stands for APNEA, BRADYCARDIA, CORONER. If you ever have a bradycardic child, check his or her airway. When kids get hypoxic, their heart rate plummets! Hypoxia is the number one reason for bradycardia in a pediatric patient, so chances are the bradycardia problem is respiratory in nature. And if it's not respiratory, it's probably respiratory. Remember the American Lung Association's motto… If you can't breathe, nothing else matters! So, if the pediatric patient is apneic, check the airway. And if the pediatric patient is bradycardic, check the airway. And if you don't check the airway, be prepared to call the coroner.

DEFG

If we expand our pediatric ABCs lesson even further, we find the next set of letters. DEFG stands for **DONT EVER FORGET GLUCOSE**! This is probably the most overlooked lab value in the pediatric population, especially with the littlest ones and the coldest ones. Now, you really know your ABCs!

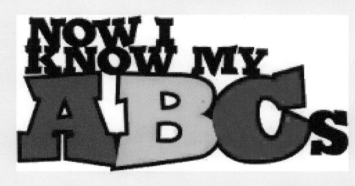

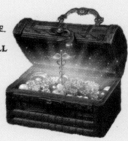

Info@PediEd.com 〰 1-888-280-PEDS (7337) 〰 PediEd.com

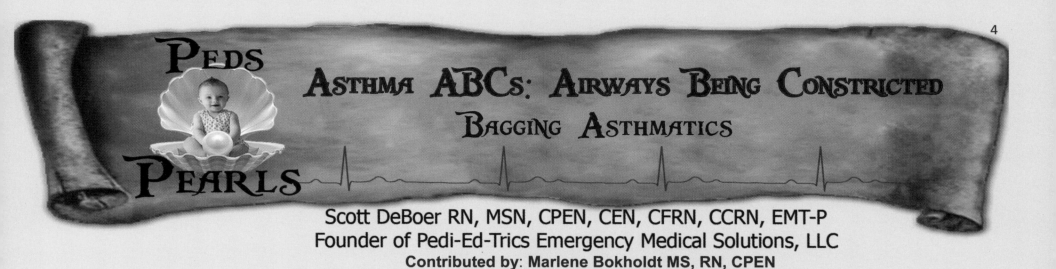

PEDS PEARLS

ASTHMA ABCs: AIRWAYS BEING CONSTRICTED
BAGGING ASTHMATICS

Scott DeBoer RN, MSN, CPEN, CEN, CFRN, CCRN, EMT-P
Founder of Pedi-Ed-Trics Emergency Medical Solutions, LLC
Contributed by: Marlene Bokholdt MS, RN, CPEN
with insights from Stu McVicar RRT, FP-C, CCEMT-P

Asthma is all about air movement (or constriction thereof). We need to consider both the anatomy and the physiology of the respiratory system, the structures, and the functions. When we talk about asthma and constricted airways, we can identify three big components:

1) Airway inflammation

2) Smooth muscle contraction

3) Secretions filling the lower airways

To better understand asthma, let's look at how those changes in the anatomy affect the physiology. We usually think about asthmatic patients having trouble with taking a deep breath. But there is another really big problem with asthma and that is the inability to exhale fully. So, what's going on inside the chest that makes asthma so bad?

Despite what you may have heard or thought, asthmatics do not generally have normal chest X-rays. Granted, they rarely have infiltrates or signs of pneumonia (unless something else is going on), but the chest X-ray of a patient with an exacerbation of asthma will tend to show lungs that are hyperinflated and therefore, hyperexpanded. That means the dark parts look darker and the arch at the diaphragm is flattened. Additionally, the great vessels are sometimes compressed (squished) resulting in decreased vascular markings. If this expanding and compressing gets bad enough, the heart is also squished and may appear long and narrow. As we all know, to stay alive, two things have to happen; Air has to go in and out and blood has to go round and round. With severe asthma, both of these may be compromised.

As you can imagine, both a flat diaphragm that is unable to help you exhale and a "squished" heart are both bad things! Remember that the problem with asthma is not only getting air in, but also getting air out!

If you are manually "bagging" your patient, chances are that you will need to **SLOW DOWN THE BAGGING** to minimize hyperinflation! Make the exhalation phase far longer than inhalation. Make it even longer if you see signs of decreased cardiac output such as pale, cool skin, weakened pulses, tachycardia, or even worse, dropping blood pressure.

If your intubated asthmatic is mechanically ventilated, you can force air in, but it may seem like it never fully comes out. If you take your patients off of the vent for a moment and watch them as they exhale, you may think that it is taking way too long before they take their next breath. So, you may need to adjust the ventilation rate to allow far more time for exhalation.

Imagine that you are assuming care of a 4-year-old asthmatic child. With all of the excitement going on, you notice that your patient is intubated and being bagged at a rate of 50 times per minute. With this seriously fast bagging rate, it should be no surprise to find all of the signs of decreased cardiac output as previously described. This child is not only on the edge of the cliff, but about to fall off! You gently take over ventilation and with SLOW bagging (i.e., a rate of 8) her condition SLOWLY starts to improve.

As you have just shown your colleagues, the asthma issue is compounded with the cardiac output issue. It is crucial to allow time for filling the heart. Your patient's recovery is very much about the cardiopulmonary interactions in this case! Bagging too fast increases the intrathoracic pressure and often affects venous return to the heart.

Normal Airway — muscle, lining

Airway in Person With Asthma — tight muscle, swelling, mucus

The best way to determine the optimal ventilator rate is to LISTEN!!! Give a breath and listen until the patient reaches the end of exhalation or at least close to the end of exhalation. Then and only then should you (or the ventilator) give another breath. Sometimes, in really bad asthmatics, you will actually have to push on their chest to get air out.

Moral of the story

Overbagging the pediatric asthmatic patient is bad. A very long exhalation phase is good. Air goes in and out… Blood goes round and round… Any variation of this is a bad thing!

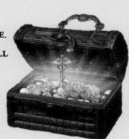

Info@PediEd.com ☏ 1-888-280-PEDS (7337) ☏ PediEd.com

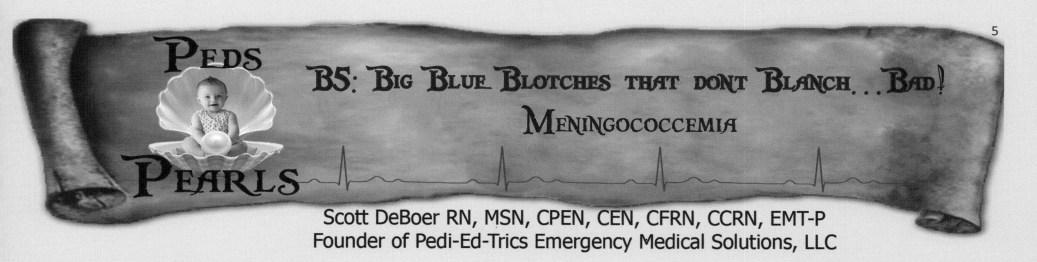

B5: Big Blue Blotches that don't Blanch... Bad!

Meningococcemia

Scott DeBoer RN, MSN, CPEN, CEN, CFRN, CCRN, EMT-P
Founder of Pedi-Ed-Trics Emergency Medical Solutions, LLC

Seizing... Stiff neck... Bulging fontanels...All of these findings should immediately bring to mind one of the most feared medical maladies: **Meningitis**. There are variations of meningitis, each worse than the next; and high on that "worse than" list is the dreaded meningococcal meningitis and/or meningococcemia (when the bug gets into the blood). This particularly troublesome form of meningitis has some classic characteristics and to help you remember what they are, just remember **B5**!

1) Big: Big random rashes (larger than 2 mm) are very possibly bad, especially if the kid looks sick.

2) Blue: Big and blue (purply-bruisy looking) rashes are very possibly bad, especially if the kid looks sick.

3) Blotches: Big blue blotches (no pattern to them) are very possibly bad, especially if the kid looks sick. Nicely formed small circular, or poxy-polka-dot rashes are one thing. Big blue blotches are another.

4)*That don't* Blanch: This is a crucial part of **B5**. When you think about blanching, think about capillary refill. If you push on your nailbed and it immediately loses color, that's blanching. (It should also pink up again very quickly indicating adequate perfusion). But, if you push down on one of the big blue blotches and it *doesn't* blanch, that's a really bad sign!

5)*Are* Bad: The symptoms above add up to meningococcemia (and possibly meningococcal meningitis). In a nutshell, that is really, really bad.

Experience tells us that most petechial (tiny red or blue/purply) rashes are not meningococcal, but, in the interest of patient care, we should consider that they all can be meningococcal until proven otherwise, *especially if the kid looks sick*.

Sometimes life's important concepts can be expressed in a few, easy to remember words. In the case of sick looking kids with rashes... **Big Blue Blotches that don't Blanch are Bad!**

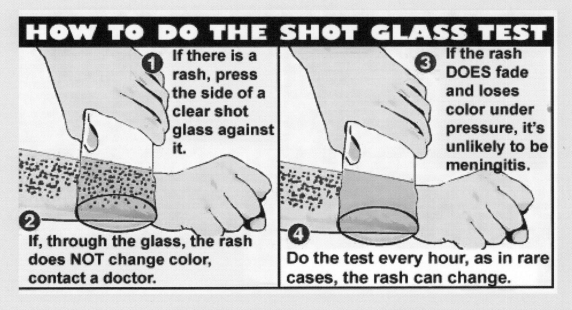

HOW TO DO THE SHOT GLASS TEST

1 If there is a rash, press the side of a clear shot glass against it.

2 If, through the glass, the rash does NOT change color, contact a doctor.

3 If the rash DOES fade and loses color under pressure, it's unlikely to be meningitis.

4 Do the test every hour, as in rare cases, the rash can change.

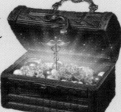

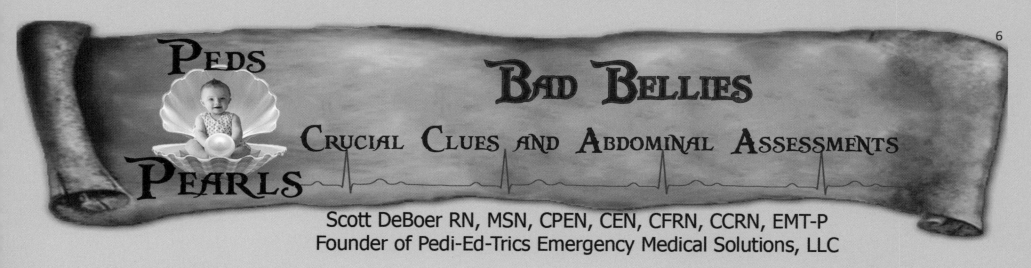

PEDS PEARLS

BAD BELLIES
CRUCIAL CLUES AND ABDOMINAL ASSESSMENTS

Scott DeBoer RN, MSN, CPEN, CEN, CFRN, CCRN, EMT-P
Founder of Pedi-Ed-Trics Emergency Medical Solutions, LLC

Bad Belly Clues

When it comes to emergencies and kids, whether from minor "owies" or major trauma, chances are pretty good that if they didn't mess up their big ol' heads, then they probably have an issue with their bellies. So, beyond CT scans (no, everyone does not need a CT scan...), what are some clinical signs that should clue you in that the kid might have a bad belly?

Kehr's sign– Shoulder pain without shoulder trauma. This is referred shoulder pain from a messed up and bleeding spleen pressing against nerves in the diaphragm. Shoulder begins with "S" and Spleen begins with "S." If they have shoulder pain <u>without</u> shoulder trauma, it might be because they were "K"icked in the belly and that's "K"ehr's sign.

Cullen's sign– Bruising around the bellybutton. The first two letters in Cullen's are "CU." If you "C" bruising around the "U"mbilicus, that's Cullen's which hints at a retroperitoneal, or back of the belly bleed. Remember, bruising doesn't happen right away, and you won't see this sign right away.

Grey-Turner's sign– Bruising on the flank. If you tell the patient to "Turn" over and you see bruising on their side (flank,) that's Grey-"Turn"er's sign which also hints at a retroperitoneal or back of the belly bleed. And again – this bruising may not be seen right away!

Seatbelt sign– Bruising along the belly where the seatbelt would be. This one is pretty self-explanatory. If the kid has horizontal bruising across the belly where the lap belt was, that's a seatbelt sign (imagine that) and hints at not only a possible belly injury, but also **Chance** fractures of the lumbar spine. You are taking a "Chance" if you only use a lap belt!

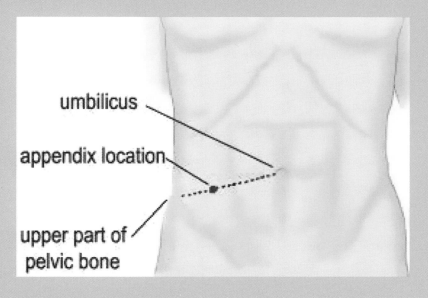

umbilicus

appendix location

upper part of pelvic bone

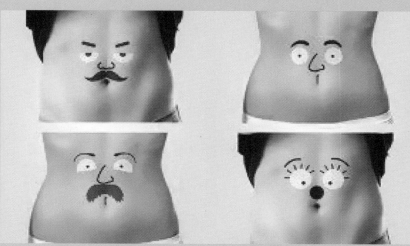

McBurney's point– Pointing to pain in the right lower quadrant. McBurney's point is located 2/3 of the distance between the bellybutton and the right iliac spine (top of the hip). Rebound tenderness (pain when you push down, but especially when you suddenly stop pushing and let your hands up) at McBurney's suggests appendicitis. There might not be a good connection here, but I like to think about *Weekend at Bernie's* (a truly classic film which somehow avoided the Oscar judges...) because an emergency appendectomy can pretty much ruin your weekend plans.

Currant jelly stool– Stool that looks like currant jelly is a sign of a possible intussusception. What we are looking for is stool mixed with blood and mucous (yuck!) Let's be honest...what does currant jelly look like? Does anyone really know? Has anyone ever actually eaten currant jelly? Not the stool, just the jelly! Strawberry jelly? Sure. Grape jelly with peanut better? Absolutely. But currant jelly? Not so much. But, if someone mentions currant jelly stool, think about intussusception.

In Conclusion...

If the kid is sick as a dog and diagnostic imaging is required, expect a call for CT and/or ultrasound. This is especially true if non-operative management for an injury is going to be done (i.e., wait, watch, and let them heal). But since not everyone needs to go to CT, when you are trying to figure out if the kid has a bad belly, repeated assessments which would include looking, listening, and feeling the belly are incredibly appropriate!

Info@PediEd.com 〰 1-888-280-PEDS (7337) 〰 PediEd.com

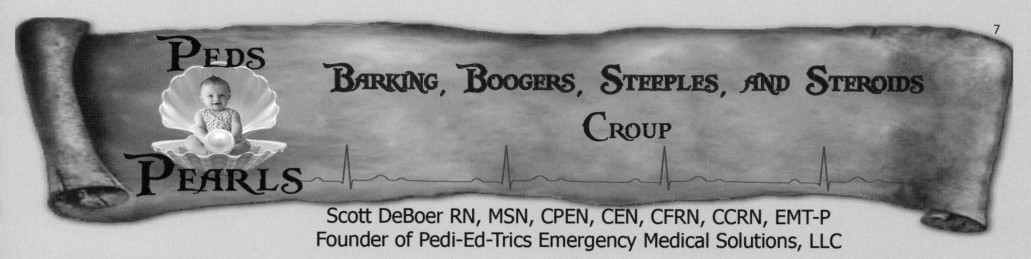

Peds Pearls

Barking, Boogers, Steeples, and Steroids
Croup

Scott DeBoer RN, MSN, CPEN, CEN, CFRN, CCRN, EMT-P
Founder of Pedi-Ed-Trics Emergency Medical Solutions, LLC

Let's Clarify

Call it a croupy cough or a barking cough; if you hear it, you know it. It's croup. And what do you do with a croupy kid? You watch 'em and that's all there is to it. Or is it? Let's clarify a few medical misconceptions and common queries.

First, remember that croup is a viral infection at the bottom of a little kid's funnel shaped airway. Like thermal injuries, an infection produces swelling, and just like smoke inhalation and with real estate, it's all about location, location, location. If that inflammation is at the bottom of the funnel shaped airway, a little swelling goes a long way. To help reinforce the importance of this concept, remember that the pediatric airway is just plain smaller. Picture an airway the size of a dime (kid) versus the size of a quarter (adult). Even a very small amount (1-2mm) of swelling is truly significant and makes a big difference in terms of air flow. If you do a neck X-ray on a croupy kid and view it upside down (the X-ray, not the kid), you will commonly see a "Steeple Sign." That is where the airway gets narrow and it resembles the top of a church steeple. But remember the start of this paragraph. The cause of the swelling is viral which means that antibiotics aren't needed, despite what many parents will expect and even request.

What can parents do in the middle of the night to help croup? 1) Take them into the bathroom, shut the door (to contain the steam and to avoid waking the other kids), and turn on the shower for a warm mist treatment. 2) What's even better from the perspective of the anxious parent? Bring the croupy cougher to the ER! Upon arrival to the ER, what we often hear is some variation of, "You are going to think I'm nuts, but 20 minutes ago, my kid was barking like a seal and now they're all better." True. What happened between the house and the ER? A combination of cool mist treatment, repositioning, and the unseen hand of a higher power beyond our knowing.

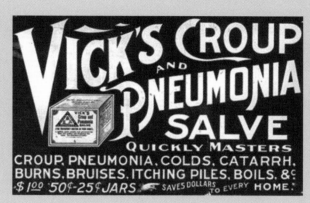

So, since it's poor form to tell parents to take their child back outside to the parking lot, what are our alternatives? Until relatively recently, we would bring out the infamous Croupette (aka the mist or croup tent). But that was then and this is now. We don't use that thing anymore. In recent years, research has shown that croup tents don't really help croup and are fraught with problems such as:

1) They don't help croup and germs love moist environments
2) The kid is always trying to get out and the Mom or Dad is always trying to get in
3) The sheets are saturated and cold which is in direct violation of another *Peds Pearl* which reminds us to keep kids pink, warm, and sweet - not cold, wet and purple.

What is the current recommendation for that mist tent if you still have one?

Take it out back, take a picture of it, and then throw it away. So, if the old croup tents are things of the past, what are we to do now? One might expect an answer like, "No worries, we will just provide blow-by cool mist." However, here's ER research at its coolest. Croupy kids were randomized into two groups. One immediately got blow-by cool mist. The other immediately got sent to the waiting room and got nothing at all. And the ones who sat in the waiting room did just as well as those who got cool mist!

But all bets are off if you have a bad crouper with stridor at rest. If the croupy cough is accompanied by high-pitched noises (most commonly on inspiration), then racemic epi (Vaponephrin) nebs are your best friend. As the neb treatment begins and the patient inhales the epinephrine, the swollen airway tissues shrink in size and breathing improves. Up until recently, however, if you gave a racemic epi, the child also automatically got admitted because of concerns about rebound edema (i.e., edema that went away and came back). Current research shows that if the kid is still sick after a few racemic epi's or requires *more* than three racemic epi's, s/he is truly sick. And what do we do with truly sick kids? Admit them or get them someplace where an appropriate level of care can be provided. And yes, it's rare, but some kids actually do get sick enough from croup to require intubation. But your patient may go home after a single racemic epi treatment if:

- The patient has one dose of steroids such as Decadron (dexamethasone or "dex") on board
- You have watched them for a few hours (2-4 post-steroids)
- They and the parents are cute and comfortable (and possibly even sleeping quietly)

Note about the steroids: IM or PO dexamethasone both work equally quickly. PO or ODT Orapred (prednisolone) may also be used if you don't have oral "dex" solution, but it requires the child taking a few days of meds at home versus one ER dose of dexamethasone.

Moral of the story

When croupy children hit the door, give them steroids. That way, even if you have to give them a racemic epi, they already have the steroids on board. The watching clock starts only if you give racemic. If they haven't had rebound after a couple of hours since the racemic epi, they are not going to get rebound. Send them home, bag the blow-by, and burn the Croupette!

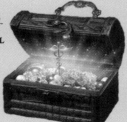

Peds Pearls™ is a registered trademark of Pedi-Ed-Trics Emergency Medical Solutions, LLC and is intended to provide accurate pediatric emergency Tips, Tricks, and Treasures for emergency medical professionals when caring for critically ill or injured children. However, always follow your medical director's specific protocols.

✂ Contact us to have Scott DeBoer or one of our other pediatric experts present at your next conference.

Info@PediEd.com 🕾 1-888-280-PEDS (7337) 🕾 PediEd.com

PEDS PEARLS

BIG HEAD, LITTLE BODY SYNDROME
IMPLICATIONS FOR MEDICAL AND TRAUMA CARE

Scott DeBoer RN, MSN, CPEN, CEN, CFRN, CCRN, EMT-P
Founder of Pedi-Ed-Trics Emergency Medical Solutions, LLC

In real estate, the key to success is location, location, location. With little kids, the key to success in many cases is head size, head size, head size. Little kids, especially those under the age of two, have a medical phenomenon often referred to as "Big Head, Little Body Syndrome." Their bigger head size makes a big difference, especially in situations related to airway management, trauma, burns, and drowning.

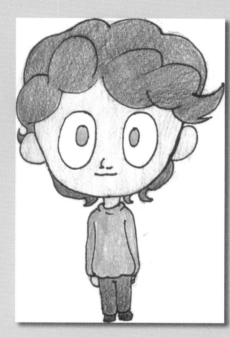

Airway: Think about placing one-year-olds with a big ol' heads (imagine Charlie Brown) flat on a spine board or sedated for a CT scan. What does their big heads do to their airways? It shoves their chins onto their chests, kinks off that flexible little kid trachea, and then, unsurprisingly, they tend not to breathe very well. Simply putting a diaper or towel under their shoulders or placing little ones under three months of age in the "Peanut" papoose (www.ossur.com) goes a long way to offset "Big Head, Little Body Syndrome" and improve airway patency.

Trauma: The purpose of spinal immobilization/restriction is to help maintain the spine in proper position. But, if the child's chin is on their chest and the cervical spine X-ray looks like a "U," that defeats the purpose of immobilization. As with the airway management suggestion above, a little padding under the shoulders, peanut papoose, or pediatric spine board goes a long way (and is often crucial) for maintaining proper trauma positioning.

Drowning: Little ones are curious creatures who, when not under general anesthesia, seem to be in perpetual motion. And unlike horses, kids don't need to be led to water. They find it on their own just fine. So, when you combine that perpetual motion with any sort of body of water (from bucket or bathtub to lake or ocean), they tend to fall in. And when they fall in, how do they fall? Head first, of course. Why? Physics says – heaviest part first, so, the culprit again is - Big Head, Little Body Syndrome.

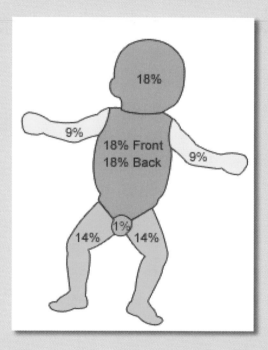

Burns: The Rule of 9's teaches us that there are two kinds of body parts: Little parts (9%) and big parts (twice that amount – 18%). In adults, "little parts" include the head and get counted as 9% of the body surface area. However, when we remember that little children have "Big Heads," they get the "big part" percentage, or 18% for their big ol' head.

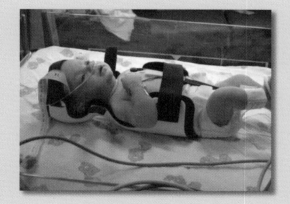

Moral of the story
In little kids who look like little kids (under 2-years-old), whether for medical or traumatic emergencies, you must remember the implications of Big Head, Little Body Syndrome!

www.ossur.com

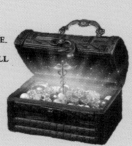

Info@PediEd.com ☏ 1-888-280-PEDS (7337) ☏ PediEd.com

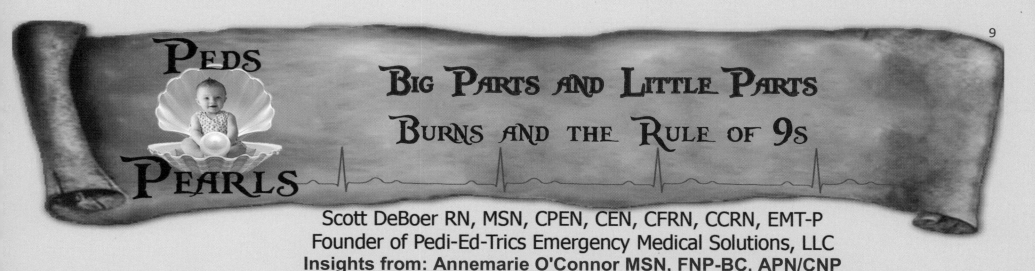

BIG PARTS AND LITTLE PARTS
BURNS AND THE RULE OF 9S

Scott DeBoer RN, MSN, CPEN, CEN, CFRN, CCRN, EMT-P
Founder of Pedi-Ed-Trics Emergency Medical Solutions, LLC
Insights from: Annemarie O'Connor MSN, FNP-BC, APN/CNP

Burnt Kids

If EMS or ER professionals have work related fears, a common and often cited element of concern is pediatric patients, or simply put, kids. And what's even worse than kids? Kids that are burned. While our initial reaction may be just to call the burn center and say that the kid is burned, or badly burned, or badly, badly burned, what they need and should expect from us during the initial phone call is a realistic approximation of the amount or percentage of body surface that is burned. So, here's our suggested way to calculate and actually remember how badly a kid is burned.

Before we can actually explore the calculation rule, there are a couple of key reminders:

1) The Rule of 9s is only a guide. It's not perfect by any means. But in the prehospital or ER arenas, it will get you in the right ballpark until the patient can arrive at a burn center.

2) Little kids, under the age of two, have "big head, little body syndrome." As a result, they get a much bigger percentage assigned for their bigger heads.

Big Parts and Little Parts

The Rule of 9s teaches that there are two kinds of body parts: Little parts and big parts. The little parts are worth 9%, hence, the Rule of 9s. Imagine that. Big parts are bigger so they get twice that amount, or 18%. In adults, "little parts" include one entire arm or the entire head and get 9%. "Big parts" are made up of two little parts, such as the anterior torso which includes the chest and abdomen, or an entire lower extremity which includes both the anterior and posterior aspects. These bigger parts get 18%. So, if the front of the chest and belly are a big part and worth 18%, how much does the entire back of the torso get? 18%. That wasn't hard, now was it?

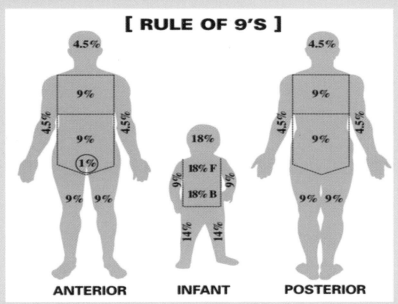

[RULE OF 9'S]

ANTERIOR   INFANT   POSTERIOR

However, remember that little children (<2-years of age) have "big head, little body syndrome" and therefore, they get 18% for their big 'ol heads. Burn centers who like caring for burns teach that little children also have "short little leg syndrome" and they technically only get 14% for their legs. However, for us in EMS or the ED where we don't take care of critically ill burn patients every day, simply remembering "big parts (18%) and little parts (9%)" is much easier and sufficient in most cases. When the patient gets to the burn center, they can more accurately assess the burn percentage using the Lund-Brower chart or other methods. They are the experts as they do this every day!

And don't worry about your math skills… If you add up all the numbers and get a negative number or a number greater than 100%, the burn unit will pay attention and usually understand. Trust me on this one!

The Math…

Example 1: A one-year-old has burns to his entire head and both arms. What % is burned? (Hint: Big Head at this age.)
- Big parts (18%) vs. little parts (9%)
- Big head (little kid with big head = 18%) and two little parts (arms) at 9% each
- 18 + 9 + 9 = Approximately 36% burn

Example 2: A 12-year-old has burns to his entire head, both arms, and the front of his chest. What % is burned?
- Big parts (18%) vs. little parts (9%)
- Big part (front of chest = 18%) and three little parts (head, both arms) at 9% each
- 18 + 9 + 9 + 9 = Approximately 45% burn

Pediatric Burn Surface Percentages…Remember:

1) Big parts vs. little parts

2) Little kids have big head, little body syndrome

3) You can always phone home (to the burn center) for help, but sometimes you just have to do the math!

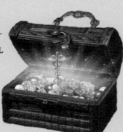

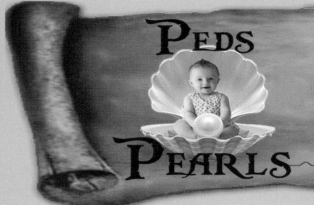

Bigger vs. Better vs. Nothing? Choosing Bag and Mask Sizes

Scott DeBoer RN, MSN, CPEN, CEN, CFRN, CCRN, EMT-P
Founder of Pedi-Ed-Trics Emergency Medical Solutions, LLC
Contributed by: Stu McVicar RRT, FP-C, CCEMT-P

Tight Situation?... Believe it or not, there have been situations when pediatric resuscitation was delayed or even withheld because "we didn't have the appropriate sized peds equipment." That is what was reported even though before, during, and after the child was crashing, an adult bag and mask were hanging on the wall less than three feet away. As you can imagine, not only is this type of occurrence a patient care nightmare, but also a malpractice case waiting to happen!

What To Do... If you find yourself in the middle of the "no-right-size-peds-equipment" nightmare, but have a larger manual resuscitator bag ("Ambu" bag) available, **use it!** Just because you have a bag that can deliver 1500 mL, <u>doesn't</u> mean you have to squeeze out all 1500 mL. Though not ideal, in a pinch, you can ventilate a small child, infant, or even a neonate with an adult bag. Even if you have the "right-sized" bag, but can't get good chest rise with it, try going up a size, as long as you <u>stop squeezing </u>once you get an adequate chest rise. One tip here is to use just your fingertips in helping control the pressure. That should be easy enough to remember… *"fingertips for compressions, fingertips for ventilations!"*

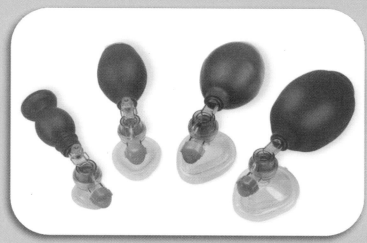

www.mercurymed.com

The same thought process applies to mask size. Though not ideal, in a pinch, you can use an adult size mask on an infant or small child and turn it 90-180 degrees until you get an adequate seal. As long as you can gently make air go in and out, it will do the job! Once again, fingertip pressure versus full body weight should be enough to maintain the seal. The goal is to get the mask to conform to the face, <u>not</u> to make the face conform to the mask.

Go Big or Go Home... With bags, masks, and laryngoscope blades, even though it may not be ideal, there may be situations where it is appropriate to go *larger*. And with ET tubes and suction catheters, though it may not be ideal, there are situations where you need to go *smaller*. In a crisis, something is certainly better than nothing. Use whatever you have that allows air to go in and out and hopefully helps keep the child alive!

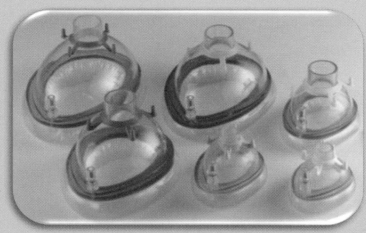

www.kingsystems.com

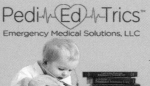

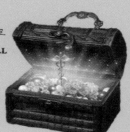

Info@PediEd.com ☏ 1-888-280-PEDS (7337) ☏ PediEd.com

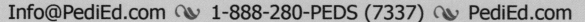

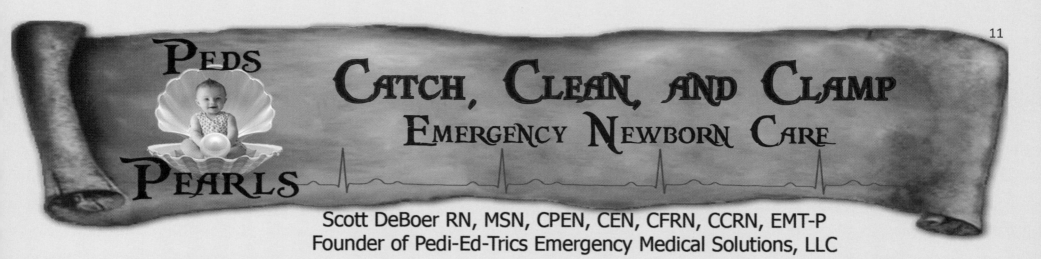

CATCH, CLEAN, AND CLAMP
EMERGENCY NEWBORN CARE

Scott DeBoer RN, MSN, CPEN, CEN, CFRN, CCRN, EMT-P
Founder of Pedi-Ed-Trics Emergency Medical Solutions, LLC

Imminent delivery... Few situations are met with the same level of apprehension and fear, even in the most experienced of medics or ED nurses such as the prospect of delivering a baby in an emergency setting. Whether this is while traveling to the hospital or even in the hospital getting to the place where they routinely do that sort of thing, most of us would agree that delivering a baby is best left to others. But remember this, if we talk with L&D nurses who like to deliver babies (and do it on a very regular basis), they will remind us that over 90% of babies do not need the sorts of things we do in the ED on a regular basis (intubation, CPR, or emergency intravenous access). In the vast majority of cases, we really need to remember three and only three things... Catch, Clean, and Clamp.

Catch: Self-explanatory. Catch the baby. For thousands of years (yes, even before you and I entered healthcare), babies were delivered successfully by people without any initials after their names. So take a breath, relax, and hold out your hands!

> Some people were dropped on their heads as babies, others were clearly thrown in the air, hit a ceiling fan, bounced off the wall, and fell out the window

Clean: Despite what we might see on TV or in the movies, babies are messy (and slippery) when they first enter this world. Cleaning off the baby will accomplish a variety of important steps:

 A – Cleaning in and around the mouth and nose helps clear the airway.
 B – Cleaning the body provides stimulation which may initiate breathing.
 C – Drying the baby will reduce the cooling effect and improve circulation.
 D – Cleaning and drying the baby helps to avoid dropping.

Newborns are slippery, cold little creatures so grab a blanket or towel (the warmer the better!) and hold on tight! But, if you drop them, what do you do? Pick 'em up. How long can they stay on the floor? What's the rule? Ask any Mom, she will tell you - five seconds!! (just like an ice cream cone).

Clamp: When you get a free minute, clamp the cord. In the past, as soon as the baby was all the way out, we frantically clamped the cord. Nowadays, many places wait at least 30-60 seconds before clamping. If the baby is sick and immediate resuscitation is required, clamp the cord and care for the baby. But, in most cute and healthy newborns, there's no huge rush to clamp the cord as long as baby and Mom are kept at the same level (i.e., baby not on the floor, Mom on the bed… that's bad!) In healthy newborns, delayed cord clamping has shown clear benefits to the babies by increasing their blood volume.

When you clamp, how close to the baby do you put the clamps? Four to five inches (8-11cm) is great. Three feet (1m) is a bit much. Leaving a little cord for the nursery to play with is truly appreciated, especially if the baby is sick. But remember the first rule of basic carpentry; "Measure twice, cut once." In our case, it's "clamp twice, cut once." If you clamp once and cut once, someone is going to bleed. So, clamp twice and cut once (between the clamps).

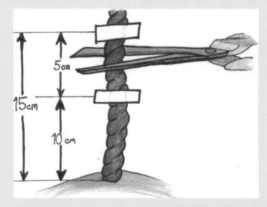

So, if Mom screams those sweet words we dread hearing..."I've gotta push!!!" Just remember "Catch, Clean, and Clamp."

Delivering babies is not...

 Baseball – **We don't catch and throw to another player!**

 Basketball – **We don't dribble after the catch!**

 Football – **We don't spike after a successful catch!**

Or even…

 Fishing – **We don't catch and release!**

PEDS PEARLS

CONSULTATIONS, CUSTODY, AND CRASHING CHILDREN

EMERGENCY PROTECTIVE CUSTODY

Scott DeBoer RN, MSN, CPEN, CEN, CFRN, CCRN, EMT-P
Founder of Pedi-Ed-Trics Emergency Medical Solutions, LLC
Contributed by: John R. Clark JD, MBA, NRP, FP-C, CCP-C, CMTE

A six-year-old African-American child presents to the emergency department in a sickle cell pain crisis. The parents relate that the child has been admitted to the hospital with the same diagnosis six times in the last year, with the last episode about two months ago. Today, it appears that in the addition to the pain, there is an acute stroke in progress with weakness on one side. Lab tests reveal a hemoglobin level of 4 gm/dL (the age adjusted normal range is around 11-14, so this is way too low!) A blood transfusion is required, but the parents absolutely forbid it due to their religious convictions.

What can you do?

It is a very challenging situation when a parent (or other legal guardian) refuses to permit a treatment that is considered essential for the child's well-being. While adult rights of self-determination go a long way in the courts, in cases that involve children, parental authority is not absolute. When a parent acts contrary to the best interests of a child, the state may intervene.

The best course of action is to work with the parents in an attempt to find a mutually-acceptable treatment plan which will safely manage the child's medical condition. But when faced with a parent who refuses to allow the care and/or transport necessary to prevent morbidity and/or mortality (e.g., seriously messed up or dead child), you might have to enlist the help of law enforcement and child protective services in order to have the child placed in temporary protective custody. (Consultation with hospital risk management and/or administration may also be necessary). If a life or limb threatening emergency exists, hospital security can intervene so that emergent evaluation and treatment can begin while other avenues are pursued.

What Should You Document?

Documentation should include the reasons why it was necessary to have the child taken into protective custody, any alternatives that were discussed with the parents, and of course, direct quotes and the names of everyone involved! If treatment was not provided, document a summary of the reasons given and the outcomes discussed – and remember names! In any case, a well-documented, detailed account of the care provided to the child is most critical. Record everything that may be necessary to protect you if a lawsuit, or even criminal charges, are ever filed.

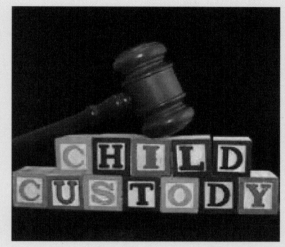

Of course, every state has slightly different laws. Generally speaking, in order to take protective custody of a child, a police officer, law enforcement official, or a physician/advanced practice provider must have <u>reasonable cause</u> to believe that a child is in <u>imminent danger</u> of suffering serious physical harm or the child's life is threatened. The temporary protective custody is for the purpose of reducing or eliminating harm and is usually only for temporary placement within a hospital or medical facility for less than 24 hours.

What Does That Mean?

That is a really fancy, legal way of saying that if the physician or advanced practice provider really feels that the child will be seriously harmed by not doing a procedure (e.g., placing a chest tube, going to the operating room for repair of a volvulus, etc.) or administering medications (blood products, antibiotics, etc.), the staff should be prepared to treat the child first and worry about the legal ramifications later. Certainly, if you have the time to consult with medical-legal experts and/or can have your supervisor or in-house legal department discuss the situation with a judge first, great. But if the child really needs to be treated, let the family and security know <u>what</u> you are going to do and <u>why</u>. Proceed with the treatment necessary, document the heck out of it, and let the hospital lawyers work out the legal matters later!

PEDS PEARLS

CRASHING KIDS WITH CONGENITAL CARDIAC CONDITIONS
CONGENITAL HEART DISEASE

Scott DeBoer RN, MSN, CPEN, CEN, CFRN, CCRN, EMT-P
Founder of Pedi-Ed-Trics Emergency Medical Solutions, LLC
Contributed by: Maria Broadstreet RN, MSN, CPNP

Why do big people drop and often die? As we know, a common problem with big people is coronary artery disease usually associated with the alphabet: Age, Blockages (aka the "Big One"), Cholesterol, and Diet. But that's big people for you. On the other hand, this alphabetic compilation is very rare for little kids. As such, it is unusual, though not impossible, to see a MI in a pediatric patient, even with those known to have a cardiac disease history. Typically in EMS or the ER, kids presenting with cardiac emergencies will fall into one of three etiologies:

1) Undiagnosed congenital heart disease (i.e., a flipped upside down and backwards heart anatomy)

2) Complications post-cardiac surgery (i.e., issues after repairing a flipped upside down and backwards heart anatomy)

3) Arrhythmias (i.e., funky heart rhythms that are too fast, too slow, or not there)

For this pearl, let's focus on children presenting with no known congenital heart disease. This is a situation which can be ruled out or in by asking about previous history, visualizing the presence or absence of a big scar on their chest, and evaluating the cardiac monitor after slapping on some ECG leads.

So, why do little ones turn purple? In the vast majority of cases, it's either respiratory issues or sepsis. But in this case, could it be something else? Absolutely! The history and presentation screams funky heart kid. (There might also be respiratory or septic issues, so expect the patient to get a full work-up until proven otherwise.)

PDA

Remember that when the baby is still inside of Mom, Mom is doing all the work. Baby's only job is to get big. And who is doing all the breathing for baby? Again, Mom. Think of fetal lungs as being like teenagers; they grow bigger, they suck up nutrients, and they have no real purpose. So, while the baby is still inside of Mom, blood, oxygenated by mom's system, gets shunted through the ductus arteriosus, a big vessel between the aorta and the pulmonary artery. In utero, this allows more blood to get sent to the body and less to the lungs. Remember, at that point in time, Mom is doing all the work of breathing and oxygenating the blood. Normally, the ductus arteriosus closes a few hours after birth, but sometimes it takes a few days or weeks (hint, hint). But sometimes, it's just ornery and we have to give the baby drugs or surgery to close it. And those solutions are just fine in the vast majority of babies with a patent ductus arteriosus (PDA).

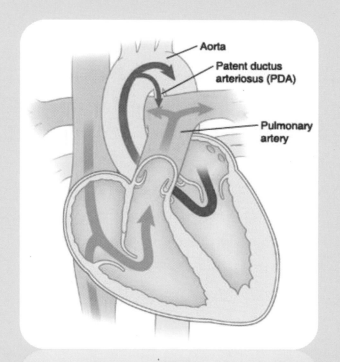

However, if you have a baby with a flipped upside down and backwards heart defect, the only thing keeping that baby alive can be blood flowing through that PDA. In these little ones with ductal dependent lesions (aka cyanotic congenital heart defects) that require the ductus arteriosus to remain open for survival, many cases can initially appear like a "normal newborn." Typically, all appears to be going well until about 1-2 weeks after birth when the ductus arteriosus closes (as it does in almost all other babies). But in these babies, the closure signals the start of a terribly frightening decline in the baby's condition. In some cases, the PDA may not close for up to six weeks post-birth; so, keep this in mind if you encounter a "few week old" baby who presents in shock or with extreme cyanosis. So... if boatloads of oxygen doesn't help bring up the sats and the child is staying purple, think CARDIAC DEFECT. (O_2 doesn't help if the oxygenated blood can't get out of the heart or to the lungs and actually can be harmful to patients with ductal dependent lesions!)

Prostaglandins

You don't have to diagnose the cardiac defect. Leave that to your friendly neighborhood pediatric cardiologist. In the emergency setting, it doesn't matter. If you have a purple little one and you are *even thinking* funky heart defect, Prostaglandins (PGE_1) are your friend. In fact, Prostaglandins are your very BEST FRIEND. In this case - the kind of friend that is going to save this kids life! Prostaglandins can keep the PDA open or reopen a PDA that's trying to close. This is hugely important as it allows blood to go here, there, and everywhere until the defect can be fixed. But, remember to watch out for Prostaglandins induced apnea and hypotension (easily fixed with intubation and/or fluids). If it turns out not to be a heart defect, but respiratory issues or sepsis - no harm, no foul - we just shut off the drip in the PICU after an echo is completed. Purple begins with "P", PDA begins with "P", and Prostaglandins begin with "P". With suspected congenital heart disease, Prostaglandins are your best friend!

CUFFED TUBES IN KIDS... CRAZY OR CORRECT?
UNCUFFED VS. CUFFED ENDOTRACHEAL TUBES

Scott DeBoer RN, MSN, CPEN, CEN, CFRN, CCRN, EMT-P
Founder of Pedi-Ed-Trics Emergency Medical Solutions, LLC

To Cuff or Not to Cuff...

For many years, it was taught that only uncuffed endotracheal tubes should be used in children. The rationale was two-fold:

1) Kids' airways are funnel-shaped and when the right size endotracheal tube just squeaked through the funnel, it created its own natural seal.

2) The pressures generated by cuffed endotracheal tubes caused tracheal ischemia and necrosis.

Both of these were true, but as the folk song goes, **"Times they are a changin'."**

First, the endotracheal tube itself continues to evolve and there are now tubes with cuffs that are "smaller/gentler" (meaning they require much lower pressure). These newer cuffed tubes don't cause the damage we used to see. Secondly, with the evolution of pediatric ventilators, improved emergency/critical care, and other significant advances in pediatric care, we are now keeping kids alive who wouldn't have survived a short time ago. These new "survivors" require more advanced respiratory management.

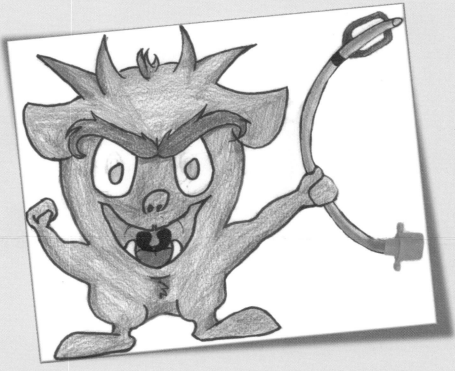

Case in point

After a horrible near-drowning incident, a kid is in ARDS and appropriately intubated. Just to barely make his chest go up and down, the patient needs ventilator pressures which seem to be something like "2,000,000 over 1,000,000" (meaning pretty much anything over 40cm H_2O). Even with the best funnel-shaped airway funnel-to-ETT fit, with these kinds of high pressures and an uncuffed endotracheal tube, the air leaks all over the place and the critically ill child may have to be extubated and reintubated with a cuffed ETT.

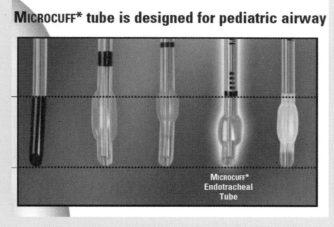

MICROCUFF* tube is designed for pediatric airway

MICROCUFF*
Endotracheal
Tube

"MICROCUFF is a registered trademark of Halyard Health, Inc. Image copyrighted by Halyard Health, Inc. Used with permission."
www.halyardhealth.com

In my transport experiences, I've seen an increasing number of pediatric ERs and ICUs that are placing cuffed pediatric ETTs. These tubes are usually ½ to 1 size smaller than the usual size for an uncuffed tube. I have also encountered an increasing number of recommendations that EDs do the same. If you don't need to inflate the cuff – great. But, if you are having trouble making air go in and out and all you have to do it put a little air into the cuff – even better! Although uncuffed tubes are still commonly used for children in the ED, in the very near future, we are likely to see the change to cuffed ETTs.

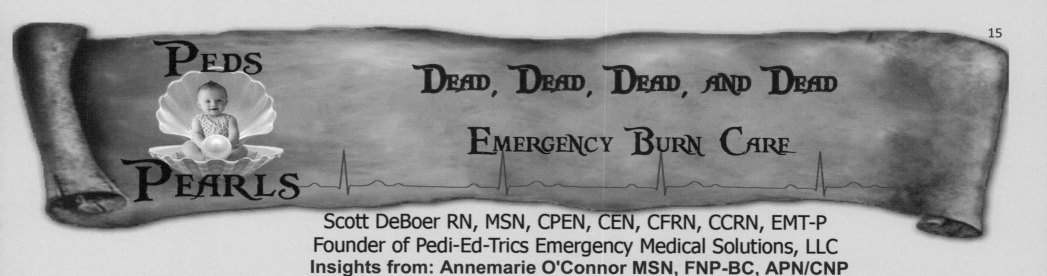

PEDS PEARLS

DEAD, DEAD, DEAD, AND DEAD

EMERGENCY BURN CARE

Scott DeBoer RN, MSN, CPEN, CEN, CFRN, CCRN, EMT-P
Founder of Pedi-Ed-Trics Emergency Medical Solutions, LLC
Insights from: Annemarie O'Connor MSN, FNP-BC, APN/CNP

It takes a special kind of person to work with pediatric patients. It also takes a special kind of person to work with burn patients. So, it figures that it takes a very, very special kind of person to work with pediatric burn patients. Even if you haven't had that experience, preparation is still important. It's better to know something and not need it, than to need to know something and not have that knowledge. Burn assessment is the first step, but pediatric burn treatment is where the time, attention, and stress are. One key bit of knowledge about burns and burn treatment is that the tissue swelling and edema associated with burns can lead to very serious consequences. And quite simply put, four of those consequences are **"Dead, Dead, Dead, and Dead!"**

Dead #1: Like many things in medical care, we start with the "A" and that stands for "Airway." Little kid airways look like funnels. They are big at the top and small at the bottom. That means that at the bottom of the funnel, at the narrowest opening through which air goes in and out, a little bit of edema can lead to a big bit of trouble. If children don't have an airway, what are they? Dead!

Dead #2: The "B" in medical care usually points us to "Breathing." Thermoregulation is an important consideration for kids and breathing. Covering a burned kid with cool, moist dressings may make you feel better, but it also makes your patient much colder, much faster. Children get cold 30 times faster if they are wet, than if they are dry. And that's if you have intact skin to help. (Remember that one of the primary functions of the integumentary system is thermoregulation. Another important function is protection against infection, a consideration for future treatment.) So, bad burns + wet dressings = a seriously cold kid. And seriously cold kids are known to have serious respiratory problems to the point where they are barely breathing. And that's a seriously bad situation because if children aren't breathing, what are they? Dead!

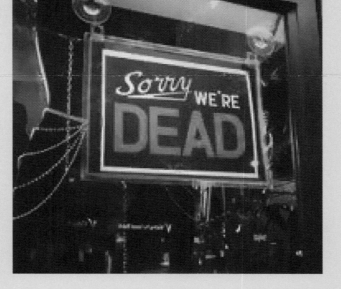

Dead #3: It should come as no surprise that after "A" and "B," we usually find the "C" and that stands for "Circulation." Managing shock and preventing renal failure in burn patients requires an amazing amount of fluid. There are guidelines like the Parkland and Brooke formulas available to help figure out just how much fluid is needed. And just as pediatric medication dosages are calculated based on weight (think "something per kilo"), burn fluids requirements are calculated based on the size of the kid and the severity of the burn. If children don't get a whole lot of fluids to maintain good circulation, what are they quickly going to become? Dead!

Dead #4: Without a doubt, burns are painful. The bigger the burn, the more the pain. That's just how it works. And in many cases, sad to say, we seriously under medicate burn patients. Most of us can only give pain meds to the extent and as often as protocols or NP/PA/Physician orders allow. But please consider this… your patients will appreciate anything and everything you can do to help control their pain. So, keep pushing the meds (or for the order to give the meds, if necessary) until your patient is comfortable (or at least not screaming). If children don't get enough pain meds, what do they wish they were? Dead!

Dead, Dead, Dead, and Dead Remember you are never alone when treating burn patients. You can always phone a friend for help at the burn center.

Info@PediEd.com ✆ 1-888-280-PEDS (7337) ✆ PediEd.com

PEDS PEARLS

FAST, FURIOUS, DROOLING, AND DYING

EPIGLOTTITIS

Scott DeBoer RN, MSN, CPEN, CEN, CFRN, CCRN, EMT-P
Founder of Pedi-Ed-Trics Emergency Medical Solutions, LLC

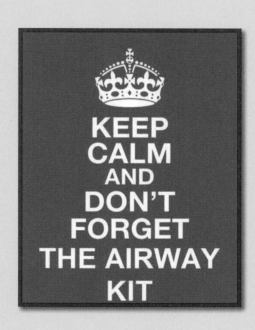

KEEP CALM AND DON'T FORGET THE AIRWAY KIT

Just as there are diseases today that weren't identified or even imagined in the not so distant past, there are diseases we had considered to be all but non-existent that seem to be making a strong and frightening comeback. From 1968 to 1992, there were fewer than 5,000 cases of pertussis reported annually in the United States. Twenty years later in 2012, the CDC reported nearly 10 times that many cases! Another disease, epiglottitis, is also making a comeback, and if that thought scares you, you're in good company!

Experienced (a polite way of saying "older") healthcare professionals remember seeing kids with epiglottitis and very often, those kids posed a significant challenge (a polite way of saying that they scared the heck out of us)! The kids were sick as a dog and at times it seemed that they were actively trying to die. Haemophilus influenzae type B (Hib) was the culprit 90% of the time. The introduction of the H. flu (Hib) vaccine dramatically reduced the number of cases of epiglottitis. But epiglottitis is still around, just with different organisms (Strep. Pneumo and others) causing the terror. Interestingly, even if the child is fully immunized, s/he still can get H. flu epiglottitis.

Epiglottitis is still an issue with three categories of patients:

1) Those under one-year of age. Be careful as presentations with these little ones can be more subtle.
2) Those who are under/not at all immunized for socioeconomic (third world countries) or personal reasons.
3) Adults, especially those of us born before the Hib vaccine. The average age of adult onset epiglottitis is now 45 years old!

And since these are "Peds Pearls," let's take a look at the classic symptoms and presentations of epiglottitis in the younger population.

Fever – Fast and Furious: Kids who have croup tend to have lots of boogers, a barky cough, and may (or may not) have a <u>mild</u> fever. Think about the last croupy child you took care of – miserable, crying, and coughing. In contrast, epiglottitis presents with a <u>fast and furious fever</u>. The kid may have looked cute at noon and then, just a few hours later, that formerly cute kid has a fever of 104°F (40°C) and a toxic FTD (fixing to die) look to them. That's not croup.

Sitting up vs. lying down: Why do kids with epiglottitis sit up? Because they can't breathe. Why do COPDers sit up? Because they can't breathe. Do COPDers ever lie down flat? Sure. When they are dead. If children with epiglottitis lie down flat it's because of only one of two reasons. Either 1) they don't have epiglottitis or 2) they are about to die.

Drooling: Why do kids with epiglottitis drool? Because they have the sore throat from Hell! It's too swollen, too tender, and they can't swallow their spit.

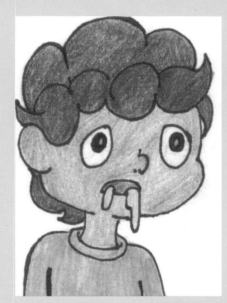

X-rays: If your patient is stable and the diagnosis is unclear, a <u>lateral</u> soft tissue neck X-ray may reveal a positive "Thumb Sign" which is indicative of a big swollen epiglottis. The key here is the stable condition and the unclear diagnosis. If all the other symptoms are screaming "epiglottitis," don't delay taking a sick kid to the OR just because X-rays aren't done. And if the kid goes anywhere, "everyone" (nurse, doc, and Mom/Dad, etc.) go with them, everywhere!

DOs and DON'Ts for Epiglottitis:

DO for EMS or ER: What do you do? Not much! Pretty much let them hang out quietly in Mom's arms. Whatever it takes to avoid making them scream and cry is a good choice. And again, anywhere they go on a road trip (X-ray, OR, etc.), everyone goes with them. And someone brings a bag-mask. Research has shown that even if a kid stops breathing from epiglottitis, bag-mask ventilation can usually be successful until a definitive airway can be obtained. While bagging is a whole lot easier than doing a cric or trache in the hallway, it's always a good idea to be prepared. Bottom line… Keep (everyone) calm and bring the emergency airway kit!

DON'T for EMS or ER: What don't you do? Lots! The biggest "no-nos" revolve around two things: 1) Don't make them cry (i.e., no IV, no labs, no ANYTHING until they are in the OR) and 2) Don't hold them down and look in their throat. Anything that makes them cry can also cause laryngospasm and make the patient lose his or her airway. Though it is commonly taught that looking with a tongue blade in their throat can precipitate them losing their airway, in reality, no cases of laryngospasm due to visualization attempts have been reported in the literature. But why push your luck and be the first one? Remember anesthesia's motto: If you make them cry, they very well might die!

Playing in the OR: First and foremost, secure the airway. Put another way, don't worry about obtaining IV access and administering IV antibiotics even in the OR until <u>after</u> the airway has been secured. In other words, if asked to prep the patient, make sure the airway is under control. Get the point? Anesthesia can put the child to sleep via mask technique, even while in Mom's arms. Who do you want to intubate this kid? Anesthesia. Where does anesthesia like to play? In the OR. In the worst and certainly rare case, a trache may be required. So, where do we like to do traches? In the OR. Ideally, evaluation and management of the airway is done in the OR and <u>only</u> when ENT and anesthesia are there and ready to play.

Prognosis & Pearls: If children get a secured airway (i.e., intubated), the mortality or death rate is less than 1%. However, if they don't have a secured airway (i.e., not intubated), the death rate can be as high as 10%. Anywhere they go, everyone goes with them. Anywhere they go, a bag-mask and cric kit goes with them. The only place they really need to go is to the OR because if you make them cry, they very well might die!

Peds Pearls

Five Tiny Trauma Triads
Bad Things Come in Threes

Scott DeBoer RN, MSN, CPEN, CEN, CFRN, CCRN, EMT-P
Founder of Pedi-Ed-Trics Emergency Medical Solutions, LLC

There is something nearly magical about the number three. There is even an ancient Latin phrase, *"omne trium perfectum,"* which roughly translates to, "Everything in threes is perfect." We hear about all sorts of things that come in threes - some good, some bad, and some that we're just not sure about. As children, we were introduced to some famous trios like the *Three Blind Mice, Three Little Pigs,* and *Goldilocks and the Three Bears.* As we grew up, many of us read about the three ghosts in the Dickens story, *A Christmas Carol,* Dumas's *Three Musketeers,* and Shakespeare's three witches in *Macbeth.* The entertainment industry seems to love things in threes, giving us such memorable trios as *The Three Stooges, My Three Sons,* and *Three's Company.* Even saying "Beetlejuice, Beetlejuice, Beetlejuice" had special qualities. As emergency medical personnel, we've seen the effects of patients being three sheets to the wind. And when it comes to pediatric trauma, there are also famous trios, or as we call them, triads.

Waddell's Triad: This classic triad is identified with trauma and is often the subject of an exam question or two. In cases where the mechanism of injury is a high velocity vehicle versus a pediatric pedestrian, these three findings comprise Waddell's triad:

1) Femur fractures – A result of the vehicle bumper hitting the child's upper leg area.

2) Chest/abdominal trauma – A result of the vehicle grill hitting the child's torso.

3) Head/spinal cord injuries – A result of the vehicle's direct impact on the child's head/neck OR as a result of the child being thrown into the air by the impact. In the latter cases, the big and relatively heavy head tends to land first, taking the brunt of the force. This third element should be anticipated, though it is not always seen in this pediatric trauma triad.

Interestingly, Waddell's triad was initially created to describe the injuries associated with _adult_ pedestrians vs. cars, but over time, it's become a pediatric trauma triad. To help remember Waddell's triad, it may be helpful to think of the injuries that result after the child "waddles" across the street and is struck by a moving vehicle. Once you identify that mechanism of injury (child vs. vehicle), simply think about the size of the child vs. the size of the vehicle and what's going to hit what.

Cushing's Triad: This is the ominous triad that appears in patients with dangerously increased intracranial pressure. In this case, think of a squished brain. There's only so much room inside the bony structure called your skull. And whether due to edema or bleeding, if there's more stuff than space, something's gotta give. The signs associated with Cushing's Triad include:

1) Blood pressure that goes way up – The increased intracranial pressure causes the blood pressure to increase as well. That's just how our body reacts as it tries to push fresh blood to the brain.

2) Heart rate that goes way down – As the brain gets squished, the brain stem gets squished as well. The result is called Cushing's reflex.

3) Respiratory rate that goes way down – This occurs for the same reasons that the heart rate goes down.

With few exceptions, if you see this triad, it's time for the family to say goodbye as it's a late and very ominous sign. If you don't get blood to your head, you are quickly going to be dead.

Beck's Triad: This is the classic triad seen in cases of cardiac tamponade. Envision a squished heart and that's pretty much what's going on. Surrounded by fluid in the pericardial sack, we find the patient exhibiting:

1) Jugular venous distention (JVD) – When the heart motion is restricted because of the seriously increased pressure of the fluid in the pericardial sac, the strength of pumping action decreases. As a result, the blood doesn't go round and round very well and we get a backup in the system. This backup causes the big, visible veins draining into the heart to get larger and more visible as the volume in those jugular veins increases.

2) Distant or muffled heart sounds – With the increased fluid in the pericardial sac surrounding the heart, the sound waves produced by the heart are affected and what we hear seems to be coming from a million miles away.

3) Narrowed pulse pressure – The restricted movement of the heart causes the systolic and diastolic blood pressures to get way too close together - never a happy thing.

When you hear Beck's, think not only of a great German beer, but also cardiac tamponade.

The Trauma Triad of Death: This is a cascading triad that if present and not quickly corrected, can result in the unfortunate and untimely death of a trauma patient.

1) Hypothermia – All too often, trauma patients are cold. Sometimes we find them that way and sometimes we make them that way. When we make those patients naked (because we can and/or need to) and then provide them with boluses of room temperature IV fluids and cold blood products, they can quickly and easily become hypothermic.

2) Acidosis – After hypothermia, the body can easily become acidotic as it attempts to compensate.

3) Coagulopathy – Last, but certainly not least, hypothermia can lead to a coagulopathic patient. This simply means that the clotting mechanisms don't work!

As you can imagine, having a multiple trauma patient who is cold, acidotic, and unable to clot is a bad combination. That's why pink, warm, and sweet is preferred to blue, cold, and dying!

Shaken Baby Syndrome: This particularly disturbing situation is typically characterized by three findings:

1) A history that isn't consistent across time (it keeps changing) and/or doesn't fit the presentation and situation by age and mechanism of injury

2) A CT scan of the head that most commonly reveals subdural bleed(s)

3) Ophthamologist confirmed retinal hemorrhages

With very few exceptions, when you see these three findings in one patient, the diagnosis is Shaken Baby Syndrome (more on this in another *Peds Pearl*).

ALL GOOD THINGS COME IN THREES

Pedi-Ed-Trics
Emergency Medical Solutions, LLC

Info@PediEd.com ❧ 1-888-280-PEDS (7337) ❧ PediEd.com

18

GOOBERS, GLUCOSE, SNOT, AND SUGAR
CSF LEAKS

Scott DeBoer RN, MSN, CPEN, CEN, CFRN, CCRN, EMT-P
Founder of Pedi-Ed-Trics Emergency Medical Solutions, LLC

Scenario... A two-year-old is in the ER after flying into the windshield of a vehicle involved in a high-speed crash. He is unresponsive, seizing, and is noted to have not only bilateral "raccoon eyes," but also clear fluid dripping from his nose. The question that comes to mind is, "How do we know if it's cerebral spinal fluid (CSF) or snot?"

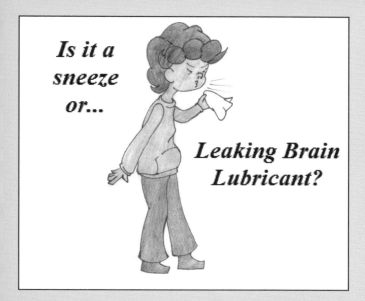

Is it a sneeze or...

Leaking Brain Lubricant?

In school, many of us were taught several assessment findings that were possibly associated with fractures of the base of the skull or basilar skull fractures. Periorbital ecchymosis (aka raccoon eyes) and bruising behind the ears (aka Battle's Sign) are two of those findings that are easily visible, though usually fairly late appearing. Hemotympanum (bleeding behind the ear drum) is another sign, but one that takes proper equipment and training to properly appreciate. And last, but certainly not least, would be the clear fluid dripping out of the ears or nose. In this Peds Pearl, let's take a look at this specific finding associated with basilar skull fractures.

So, what is up with fluid dripping out of the ears or nose? If it's clear fluid dripping out of the kid's ears, chances are it's something bad. Nothing good that's clear drips out of a kid's ears after trauma. So that one's pretty easy… clear + ear = CSF. But out of the nose, especially with crying or other confounding factors, something dripping and clear might simply be tears, snot, boogers, or mucous. And how do you tell if it's something needing a tissue or something much more serious, like CSF, meaning they get antibiotics, imaging, and possibly a trip to the OR?

Glucose test: The usual sugar level of snot (aka goober glucose level) is very low (generally less than 10). This is way lower than CSF glucose (usually 40-70) or blood glucose (around 70-100 or more). There are a couple ways you can test it for glucose: 1) *Taste it*. Downright gross and not recommended! *2) Dip it*. Do an Accucheck, Glucometer, whatever you want to call it, but definitely dip it. If it tests positive for more than just a little bit of glucose (more than 30), that fluid is possibly CSF. Remember, though, that because of the overlap of the "normal ranges," this is really only checking for "any glucose" versus testing for an actual amount of glucose. The reason that this does not work so well with blood mixed with CSF is because blood <u>and</u> CSF should always have a significant amount of glucose and therefore, they should always have a higher glucose level than normal nasal drainage. This is <u>not a perfect test</u> by any means. But, if you have little or no glucose in the clear fluid, chances are it's NOT CSF. If you have more than a little glucose, you really should do further testing to rule out a CSF leak.

Salt test: The chloride level of blood is normally 96-106. In comparison, CSF normally has a level of 122-128. That's a significant difference. So, in this case, testing bloody or blood-tinged drainage can be more meaningful. Here again, there are a couple ways you can test bloody secretions for increased chloride (and thus likely, CSF): 1) *Taste it*. Downright gross and not recommended! But if your patient is awake and communicating with you after the trauma and complains of a salty taste in his or her mouth, it could be CSF "nasal drainage" going down the back of the throat. 2) *Send it to the lab*. If the levels are much higher than normal (greater than 110), you really should do further testing to rule out a CSF leak.

Halo test: After significant trauma, fluid from the nose or ears, clear or otherwise, is potentially CSF or something (like blood) potentially mixed with CSF. So, how do you tell? In school, we were taught about the infamous "halo test." This meant that when you placed blood (mixed with CSF) onto a gauze pad or pillowcase, the CSF would separate from the blood and create a pretty "halo sign." And does it happen? Sure, but you also get the "halo sign" when blood is mixed with *tap water, tears, saline, or snot*! So, there's got to be a better way.

Beta-2 transferrin test: If you <u>really</u> want to know if it's CSF or snot, this is the confirming and single best lab test. Beta-2 transferrin is a protein that is found nearly exclusively in CSF and <u>not in snot</u>. The lab can remind you of the collection process (it's easy, but the specimen must be refrigerated immediately). However… the issue is that the test, in some laboratories, takes up to 4-days to get a result.

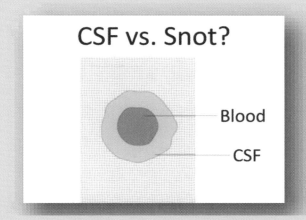

CSF vs. Snot?

Blood

CSF

In Summary... The halo test is a good answer on many written tests, but not so much in real life. Glucose and chloride levels aren't perfect, but they are a really nice and easy way to determine whether further testing should be done. And if you really want to know if it's CSF or snot, Beta-2 transferrin is where it's at!

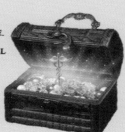

Info@PediEd.com 📞 1-888-280-PEDS (7337) 📞 PediEd.com

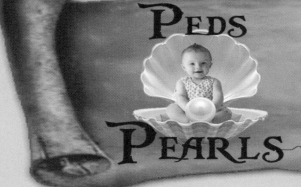

19

Peds Pearls

Guns, Drills, Bones, and Babies
Intraosseous Access: The Basics

Scott DeBoer RN, MSN, CPEN, CEN, CFRN, CCRN, EMT-P
Founder of Pedi-Ed-Trics Emergency Medical Solutions, LLC
Insights from: Teri Campbell RN, BSN, CFRN and Karen Hust RN, MSN, CEN

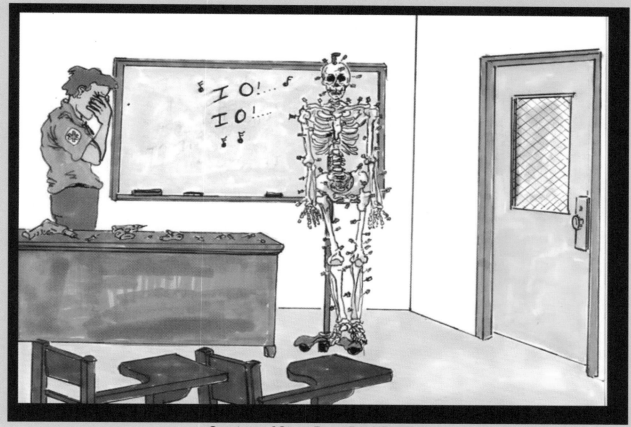

Courtesy of Steve Berry BA, NREMT-P
www.iamnotanambulancedriver.com

The Times They Are A Changin'

Many experienced practitioners remember when intraosseous (IO) vascular access, or placing a needle into the bone, was only for children and really only for children in full arrest. However, that certainly is not the case anymore. Now, intraosseous access is used for patients of all ages from babies to big people, and not just for conditions of full arrest, but for a wide variety of situations from elective procedures in fully awake patients to the most critical resuscitation attempts. Yes, as the song goes… "the times they are a changin'." So, let's take a few moments to review some of the basics!

Age: Can you place IO access into an 88-year-old? Absolutely. Can you place IO access into an 8-year-old? Absolutely. Can you place IO access into an 8-day-old? Absolutely. IO access is not just for children anymore.

Sites: Do you have to place IO access into the tibia? No. Depending on the age and device, there are now several other FDA approved IO access sites including the proximal tibia, distal tibia, distal femur, and the humerus. IO access is not just for tibias anymore.

Time: How long can you leave an IO device in place? Most IO access device manufacturers follow the US FDA recommendations of limiting the IO use to 24 hours. (In Europe, local recommendations go up to 48 hours.) And let's be honest, that should be enough time. Even on a weekend, even in more remote areas, someone can get some sort of access within 24 hours. So yes, IO access for up to 24 hours, if it's working and you need it, is still the recommendation. IO devices don't automatically need to be removed within a few hours anymore.

Devices (aka Toys): What started with bone marrow aspiration needles (Cook or Jamshidi) has now evolved into guns and drills. The traditional "twist and pop" needles are still out there and they still work, but now there are more choices. The Bone Injection Gun (aka "The Bone Gun" – www.ps-med.com) and the EZ-IO (aka "The Bone Drill" – www.teleflex.com) have made placement of an IO even faster and easier than ever. IO access isn't just with the old bone marrow aspiration needles anymore.

Meds: What drugs can you give via the IO route? Easy. With the exception of chemotherapy medications, pretty much everything that can be given IV can also be given via the IO route. And as an added bonus, meds given by the IO route reach the central circulation just as fast as those given by way of a central line. That means all ACLS/PALS resuscitation meds, antibiotics, analgesics, sedatives, blood products, etc. can be given through an IO device! And we know from actual experience that even in some of the most extreme situations, from rapid sequence intubation (RSI) on an expressway to general anesthesia of pediatric trauma patients in an OR, medications have been delivered via the IO route! As with any vascular access, IO access should be assessed for patency prior to any medication or fluid administration to decrease the likelihood of extravasation. And special caution should be used with hypertonic fluids and vesicants. IO access isn't just for resuscitation meds anymore.

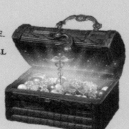

Pedi-Ed-Trics
Emergency Medical Solutions, LLC

Info@PediEd.com 〰 1-888-280-PEDS (7337) 〰 PediEd.com

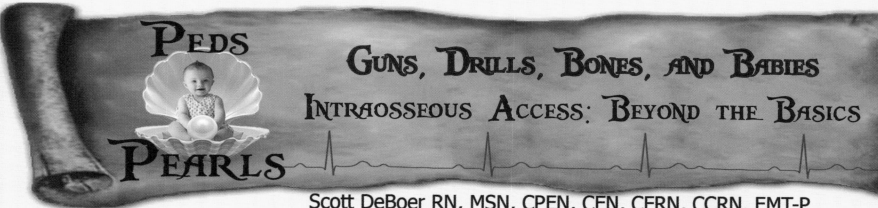

20

GUNS, DRILLS, BONES, AND BABIES
INTRAOSSEOUS ACCESS: BEYOND THE BASICS

Scott DeBoer RN, MSN, CPEN, CEN, CFRN, CCRN, EMT-P
Founder of Pedi-Ed-Trics Emergency Medical Solutions, LLC
Insights from: Teri Campbell RN, BSN, CFRN and Karen Hust RN, MSN, CEN

Many experienced practitioners remember when intraosseous (IO) vascular access, or placing a needle into the bone, was only for children and really only for children in full arrest. However, that certainly is not the case anymore. Now, intraosseous access is used for patients of all ages from babies to big people, and not just for conditions of full arrest, but for a wide variety of situations from elective procedures in fully awake patients to the most critical resuscitation attempts. Yes, as the song goes… "the times they are a changin'." So, let's take a few moments to review beyond the basics!

Complications: Current research shows that if you prep the site before you insert the IO access and take it out when you don't need it anymore, the rate of serious complications is actually less than 1%. But as you can imagine, anytime you put a needle into someone (bone, muscle, or vein), there are serious potential complications including infections, infiltrations, and compartment syndrome. As such, it is extremely important to regularly monitor the site and the surrounding tissues for signs of swelling or other unexpected events. But happily, the incidence of complications are far less than urban legends would suggest. IO access isn't fraught with danger anymore (and probably never was).

Pain (1): Sounds painful… Does it hurt? Absolutely. You are placing a big ol' needle into your patient's bone. Of course it hurts. But interestingly, if you review the published research and talk to awake "volunteers" who have had this done, the pain associated with IO insertion is not nearly as bad as you would imagine. Most describe the insertion pain as being a 2/10 or about the same pain as having a large-bore peripheral IV placed (just without the digging and probing). Some practitioners, when placing an IO device in an awake patient, will routinely inject lidocaine to numb both the skin and then the periosteum (outside of the bone). IO insertion doesn't need to be painful anymore.

Pain (2): So, when or why do the IO devices really hurt? The answer is simply this… the pain is experienced when the pressure inside the bone changes. On the inside of your bones, there are pressure receptors and when you pull out bone marrow or push in fluids or meds, it's anything but pleasant. So, to aid in this issue, device manufacturers and various healthcare centers have set recommendations for an initial (IO) dose of lidocaine (a standard dose for adults vs. "something per kilo" for kids). There now are several facilities that have even created color-coded charts to provide the suggested amounts for saline flushes and lidocaine administration. IO placement itself is not that painful, but pulling out marrow or pushing in fluids and/or meds can really hurt. The actual removal of the IO is generally not painful. So, with some planning and some lidocaine, using your IO device doesn't have to be very painful anymore.

PURPOSE

This procedure describes a process for nursing and/or pharmacy personnel* to administer lidocaine through an intra-osseous catheter to decrease infusion related pain in a conscious patient. IO insertion may cause mild pain in conscious patients but IO infusions may cause severe discomfort. Lidocaine is meant to be used as an anesthetic and not as analgesia.

Broselow Color	Weight (KG)	0.5 mg/kg Lidocaine (mg)	20mg/ml Lidocaine (ml)	Normal Saline (ml)
Grey	3	1.5	0.08	0.92
Grey	4	2	0.1	0.9
Grey	5	2.5	0.13	0.87
Pink	6-7	3.4	0.17	0.83
Red	8-9	4.25	0.21	0.79
Purple	10-11	5.25	0.26	0.74
Yellow	12-14	6.5	0.33	0.67
White	15-18	8.25	0.41	0.59
Blue	19-22	10.37	0.52	0.48
Orange	24-28	13	0.65	0.35
Green	30-36	16.5	0.83	0.17

This table represents approximate dosing based Broselow's weight breakpoints.

For **PEDIATRIC** patients who may or are able to perceive pain after the IO device is placed and position has been confirmed and secured.

CONTRAINDICATED in pediatric patients with acute seizures or history of non-febrile seizures.

1. May give 0.5 mg/kg (Max 20mg) of 2% lidocaine (without preservatives or epinephrine) IO as a slow bolus
2. Diluted with Normal Saline to a total volume of 1 ml. (See table below)
3. Wait at least 30 seconds then flush with 5mls of normal saline.
4. If necessary, step 1 may be repeated as needed to maintain anesthetic effect.
(Do NOT exceed 3mg/kg/24hr)

Chart courtesy of Stacie Hunsaker RN, MSN, CEN, CPEN

Bottom line

You shouldn't avoid the IO route anymore if: 1) you have a baby or a big person, 2) you have some IO access points available, 3) you need vascular access that works just as fast as a central line does, 4) you need access that can be used for just about every sort of medication or fluid, and 5) you need it quickly and relatively easily with few potential complications. IO access is not just for crashing children anymore!

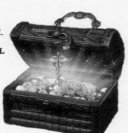

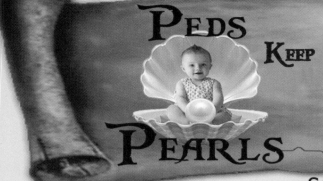

21

PEDS PEARLS

Keep 'em Pink, Warm, and Sweet...Everything Else is Fluff
Pre-Transport Pediatric Priorities

Scott DeBoer RN, MSN, CPEN, CEN, CFRN, CCRN, EMT-P
Founder of Pedi-Ed-Trics Emergency Medical Solutions, LLC

Little Kids, Big Stress

For the most part, EMS and ER professionals are happiest and most comfortable when they are taking care of "big people." You can give an ER nurse a 300 kg patient complaining of shortness of breath while smoking a cigarette through a trache and the nurse won't bat an eye. You can ride with EMS professionals as they roll up to the scene of an adult patient with a "big ol' knife" stuck in their chest and it might seem just like another routine call. On the other hand, most of those same healthcare professionals experience a high level of stress when caring for kids. And when it comes to kids, the smaller the child, the higher the stress.

When I first started playing flight nurse, a brilliant neonatologist taught me his two priorities for babies and transport:

1) Keep 'em pink, warm, and sweet.

2) Everything else is fluff.

His theory was that however well you taped the endotracheal tube or the IV, the accepting ICU was going to redo it upon arrival. So, why mess with it? Just keep the kid pink, warm, and sweet. So now, and for over twenty years, I have been passing on his pediatric pearl of wisdom to nurses, RTs, medics, and docs around the world.

Pink: Keep them pink. With little ones in EMS or the ER, you can generally give them as much or as little oxygen as needed to maintain oxygen saturations in the 94%-99% range. If they are known to have a complex cyanotic congenital heart disease (sometimes referred to as a "not fully fixed funky heart kid"), they will never be pink and will never have normal sats until their heart is fully fixed. On the rare occasion that you are caring for one of these cardiac kids, particularly those with single ventricle anatomy, you have to be careful as giving too much oxygen can seriously mess them up. Most little kids in the ER do not have a funky heart disease and are not COPDers, so go nuts... give them oxygen!

Warm: Keep them warm. In the ER, the sicker the patient, the more we keep them naked. We want to see their injuries. We want to see their perfusion. And even though we don't want to, we make people cold! So, look at what you need to look at, then do your patient a favor and cover them up. Do this not only for privacy, but also to avoid hypothermia. Remember, when little ones get cold, not only do they get sicker, but they can get bradycardic or stop breathing just because they are cold. So, cover the little ones up with warm blankets and don't forget to cover their big ol' heads. Do what you need to do. See what you need to see. Then cover them up!

Sweet: Make them act sweet. This is a two-fold effort. First, check their blood sugar. Do this when you initially see them and then, at the very least, again before they leave with the transport team. Do a finger-stick, heel-stick, or something-stick for sugar. Little ones, when stressed, use up their sugar quickly, so make sure they stay sweet. Second, make them act sweet. If they appear to be (or have every reason to be) in pain, give them something for pain (morphine, Dilaudid [hydromorphone], ketamine, fentanyl, etc). If they are intubated and don't want to be intubated, there are lots of drugs out there to make them not mind the fact that they are intubated.

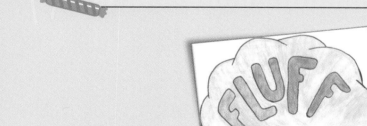

Pink, Warm, and Sweet - That's the key. And when in doubt, remember, you can always phone home (to the baby ICU or peds ICU for help). But with few exceptions... everything else is fluff!

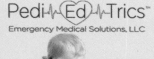

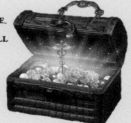

Info@PediEd.com ☎ 1-888-280-PEDS (7337) ☎ PediEd.com

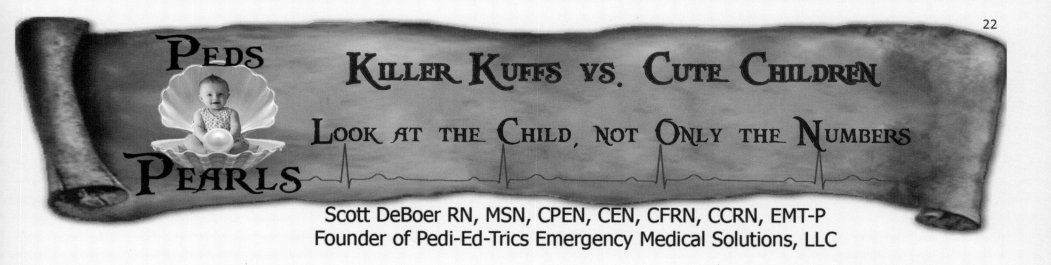

22

KILLER KUFFS VS. CUTE CHILDREN
LOOK AT THE CHILD, NOT ONLY THE NUMBERS

Scott DeBoer RN, MSN, CPEN, CEN, CFRN, CCRN, EMT-P
Founder of Pedi-Ed-Trics Emergency Medical Solutions, LLC

It's Inevitable… If you put a bunch of nurses or medics together in any sort of social gathering (especially if alcohol is involved), within just a very few minutes, we <u>will</u> start telling "war stories." So here's one of my favorite (completely true) pediatric transport tales.

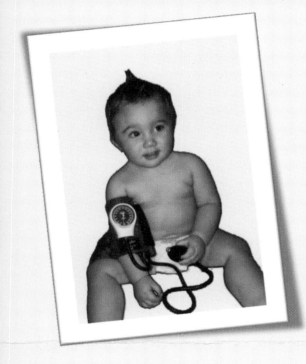

All you are told by dispatch is that the call is from a community hospital pediatric floor. They report having a two-year-old child in a "hypertensive crisis of unknown origin" and they are about to start infusing Nipride (nitroprusside). The accepting pediatric ICU attending physician tells the dispatcher … *"GO, GO, GO! Something's not right and we need to go figure out what's wrong with this kid."*

Upon arrival on the general peds floor, you are presented with the following information:

- 2-year old previously healthy child

- Admitted for asthma exacerbation and placed on q2 hours nebs

- Pediatric ICU and transport team called because of a systolic BP of 240

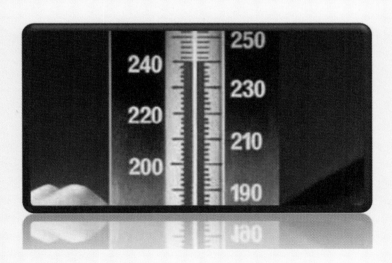

When you make your initial "Sick or Not Sick" doorway assessment, you see a really cute kid in no apparent respiratory distress. A more thorough assessment of the child reveals the following:

- A really chunky kid

- Positive "Sitting up and eating Jello" sign

- Nurse programming the IV pump to begin the Nipride infusion

- Still no apparent respiratory distress or other signs of general "badness"

- A blood pressure cuff that appears to be way too small for the aforementioned really chunky kid

Is it possible this kid is in hypertensive crisis? Sure, but is it likely? Absolutely not. How often have you seen kids in hypertensive crisis? (Hint: Never or certainly not very often are the expected answers). More importantly, are kids in true hypertensive crisis likely to be exhibiting a positive "Sitting up and eating Jello" sign? Probably not.

So, what was the issue? Small cuff and big kid. If the cuff doesn't fit the kid, the numbers don't fit. A cuff that is too small will give you numbers that are too high and vice-versa! After placement of a correct size cuff (2/3 of upper arm), we were relieved to find the BP completely normal. So… did we still transport this kid? Absolutely! Why? They were going to kill him!

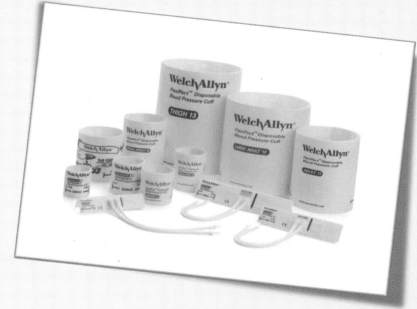

When in doubt… Look at the patient, not just the numbers. In the case of blood pressure readings, the cuff must fit the kid to get accurate numbers!

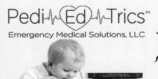

PEDS PEARLS™ IS A REGISTERED TRADEMARK OF PEDI-ED-TRICS EMERGENCY MEDICAL SOLUTIONS, LLC AND IS INTENDED TO PROVIDE ACCURATE PEDIATRIC EMERGENCY TIPS, TRICKS, AND TREASURES FOR EMERGENCY MEDICAL PROFESSIONALS WHEN CARING FOR CRITICALLY ILL OR INJURED CHILDREN. HOWEVER, ALWAYS FOLLOW YOUR MEDICAL DIRECTOR'S SPECIFIC PROTOCOLS.

✕ CONTACT US TO HAVE SCOTT DEBOER OR ONE OF OUR OTHER PEDIATRIC EXPERTS PRESENT AT YOUR NEXT CONFERENCE.

Info@PediEd.com 🕻 1-888-280-PEDS (7337) 🕻 PediEd.com

23

PEDS PEARLS

WHEN THUNDER ROARS, GO INDOORS!
LIGHTNING INJURIES

Scott DeBoer RN, MSN, CPEN, CEN, CFRN, CCRN, EMT-P
Founder of Pedi-Ed-Trics Emergency Medical Solutions, LLC
Contributed by: Daniel Griffin AS, CCEMT-P

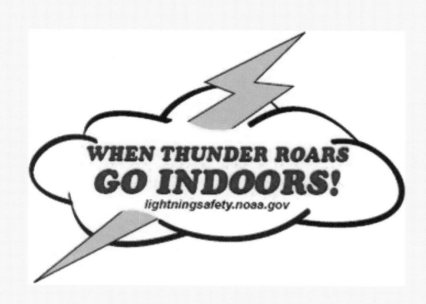

The message from a public safety campaign produced by the National Weather Service urges children and adults to go indoors when they hear thunder; indeed, that is great advice! Lightning kills approximately 55 people each year in the United States with Florida being the state with the most reported injuries (don't let Disney know).

As a general rule, only 10% of the lightning we see results in what we can call "strikes." Yes, only one out of ten lightning bolts go from cloud to ground, with 90% moving from cloud to cloud. Lightning will strike the tallest, pointiest, most isolated object within a 50 yard radius of the last branch of the lightning. Lightning can strike more than 5 miles away from the center of a storm and the odds of getting struck by it are 1 in 700,000. Most injuries occur while participating in outdoor activities, be it at work or play. Thus, if you are indoors while reading this and a thunderstorm is occurring outside, the chance that you will be struck by lightning is very slim indeed. So, by all means, continue reading the following tips, safe in the knowledge that you will be able to share this peds pearl of wisdom with others!

Prevention: Teach children (and adults!) that when they hear thunder or see lightning, they should go inside an enclosed building with solid walls and closed windows. An enclosed vehicle with a hard roof and windows rolled up will provide a safe refuge as well. More importantly, teach them **not** to take refuge under a tree, an open bus stop, in a tent, or near open bodies of water. If you are stuck in an open area, good luck! Seek shelter as soon as possible and remain sheltered until the storm has completely passed. Most importantly, pay attention to your surroundings!

Injuries: Those patients who are lucky enough to be conscious after a lightning strike will likely survive. However, the cardio-respiratory effects from a lightning strike may be devastating. Lightning can act as the "mother of all defibrillators" and put the heart into asystole. Even if the heart returns to a normal, actively beating state, the patient may still need prolonged ventilatory support after the initial resuscitation in order to survive. This is due to the electrical damage to the respiratory centers of the brain that can occur. Temporary EKG changes are not unusual in victims who do survive (Not surprising after being struck by hundreds of millions of volts of lightning!) Patients may also exhibit signs and report symptoms reflecting injuries to both the central and peripheral nervous systems such as dilated pupils despite the absence of any head injury. Patients may suffer traumatic injuries from the contact with lightning such as sudden and severe muscle contractions and should receive spinal immobilization per trauma protocols. Many victims receive superficial external burns and we can expect to discover more occult internal injuries (rupture of tympanic membranes, confusion, amnesia, cardiac injuries) after thorough assessment and testing.

Assessment and Treatment: Assessments are no different than with any other type of injury with one large exception, **multiple casualty incident (MCI) triage!** Patients in a MCI who are apneic or in cardiopulmonary arrest might appropriately be tagged "black," aka dead. But in cases of a lightning strike, patients who are unresponsive, apneic, or in cardio-pulmonary arrest should be tagged "red" and treated first! This is because those who arrested post-lightning strike did not suffer an MI due to the usual causes related to long term conditions and behaviors. Instead, they received a massive defibrillation from the high voltage lightning strike. So, if they had good hearts to begin with, and if resuscitation is promptly initiated, they might actually have a good chance of coming back to the world of the living! Beyond this, people who are awake and alive are awake and alive. After caring for the most severely ill or injured, any remaining patients should be triaged as per other mass casualty systems (START, JumpSTART, etc.).

Scene Safety: We cannot over emphasize the need to be aware of your surroundings in the out-of-hospital environment. When treating a patient outside during a storm, provide basic life support and move the patient inside an ambulance or building to prevent additional injuries to rescuers from lightning. If you think lightning will not strike twice in the same place, you may be dead wrong!

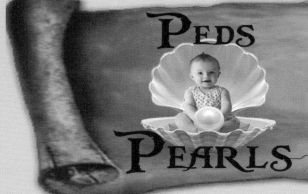

24

ALLEGATIONS AND ALGEBRA?
MEDICATION MALPRACTICE

Scott DeBoer RN, MSN, CPEN, CEN, CFRN, CCRN, EMT-P
Founder of Pedi-Ed-Trics Emergency Medical Solutions, LLC

It is said that are always two sides to any story and medical malpractice cases are no exception. The plaintiff's side is saying somebody screwed up. The defense's side is saying that everyone did the best they could and there is no fault to be assigned. While those two sides appear to be diametrically opposed, the truth may in fact lie somewhere in between, or the fault may rest with a third side of the story. So, perhaps we should say that there are always *at least* two sides to every story.

In the medical-legal arena, expert witnesses are called on to provide testimony as to what might have happened or what should have happened. Many expert witnesses have testified for both plaintiff and defense attorneys and the common thread is the pursuit of truth, whether it points to an avoidable error in judgement or action, or the conclusion that the healthcare providers did all that could be expected of them. Sometimes, the expert witness finds the third side of the story. Let's explore one such case.

Scenario...

A critically ill child was being treated in the emergency room and a peripheral IV (PIV) was successfully placed in the patient's foot. The nursing documentation indicated there was no swelling or signs of complication and that the site flushed easily. Prior to transferring the patient to a pediatric ICU, the PIV was capped and an intraosseous line placed into the tibia. During the short transport, the IO stopped functioning, the kid kept crashing, and the team started a dopamine infusion using the previously capped PIV site.

On arrival in the PICU, the child's foot was noted to be seriously swollen and nasty looking, so, the peripheral IV site was discontinued and a central line was inserted. The swollen and nasty looking foot later required extensive plastic surgery. Throughout the chart, it was assumed that the cause of the foot injury was the transport team's administration of dopamine into the "presumed to be infiltrated" peripheral IV.

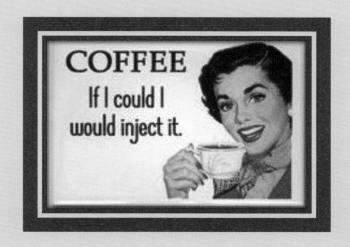

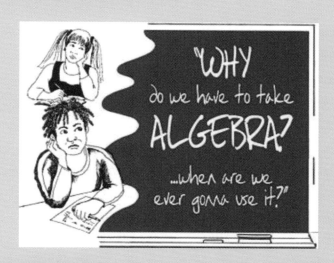

Here's where the story gets really interesting and where the allegations meet the algebra. According to the documentation, the small child only received dopamine through the PIV site for 4-minutes prior to arrival in the PICU – at which time a central line was immediately placed. Something didn't add up. Time to do the math. Exactly how many milliliters of dopamine were given in the very short time that the PIV was being used? Using the infusion rate (mcg/kg/min) and the concentration (mg/mL) and the documented infusion time, the calculations revealed that the child received 0.08mL during the four minutes of PIV dopamine infusion. (Flashback to the documentation regarding the initial placement of the PIV and the flush that went in without incident). Given that the line was placed and flushed per standard procedures, does it make sense that less than 0.1mL of dopamine would cause a foot to be swollen and seriously messed up? Probably not.

So what would make sense? Was there a third side of the story that would reveal what most likely happened? Deeper examination of the nursing documentation revealed a single entry regarding the administration of a dose of IV calcium (big red flag!) It was specifically noted to have been pushed by the ER physician (big red flag!) using the PIV prior to the time that the intraosseous line was placed into the tibia. Could the calcium that the physician pushed prior to transport cause the foot to be swollen and seriously messed up? Absolutely!

Moral of the story

We can get sued for pretty much anything. And although we've been told many, many times, it bears repeating. Good documentation is your very best defense in the event the care that you provided gets questioned. As a nursing expert, it's a great feeling to do the detective work, to find in the ER nurse's documentation that one short note about the physician pushing calcium, and to be able to establish that the nurses in question did a really great job with a really sick kid!

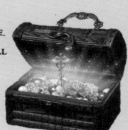

25

PEDS PEARLS

DOSES AND DECIMALS
MEDICATION MALPRACTICE

Scott DeBoer RN, MSN, CPEN, CEN, CFRN, CCRN, EMT-P
Founder of Pedi-Ed-Trics Emergency Medical Solutions, LLC

Little Ones Get Little Doses

If it looks like the tube is way too big of a tube, it *probably is* way too big. If it sounds like way too much fluid, it *probably is* way too much fluid. And… if it seems like a big person dose of a drug, it *probably is*, and that means it *is not* the correct dose for a little one.

Several years ago, there was a medical malpractice case involving a two-week-old baby who got admitted for management of MRSA. Now, how a two-week-old gets MRSA is a whole other issue, but such is life. Vancomycin is very commonly administered to help treat MRSA. Many nurses know that the big people dose of "Vanco" is 500mg to 1000mg IV. It comes premixed in a 100mL or 250mL bag and is ready to infuse. So, big people Vancomycin dosing and administration is easy. They either get 500mg or 1000mg every 12 hours. With children, however, it's not so easy. With kids, everything is weight based and usually ordered as "something per kilo." The recommended pediatric dose is 10-15 mg/kg.

The order for this 5kg infant was for 10mg/kg of Vancomycin every 12 hours - an appropriate order. But the two-week-old infant received 500mg per dose. (Hint: Does that sound like too much?) The child received <u>three</u> adult sized doses of Vanco before the decimal point error was noted. That's 10X the appropriate dose… Not once, not twice, but three times!

Vancomycin Injection, USP

500 mg

Single-Dose Container **100 mL** Iso-osmotic

Sterile Nonpyrogenic

With those facts established, the issues in question included:

❖ "How often is Vancomycin given to a two-week-old infant?"
 ➢ "Rocephin (ceftriaxone) all the time. Vancomycin not so much."

❖ "Should the fact that this was apparently an adult dose have caught the attention of the nurses?"
 ➢ "Yup. Think about it. It only makes sense that if the patient was much, much smaller, the doses should also get smaller."

❖ "Should the fact that the medication came premixed have caught the attention of the nurses?"
 ➢ "Yup. Very few IV antibiotics (or any medication) come premixed for pediatric patients."

❖ "Should the fact that the medication came in a 100mL bag have caught the attention of the nurses?"
 ➢ "Yup. Adults get that much fluid for antibiotics. 2-week-old babies, not so much. Again, smaller patient, smaller amount of fluid."

❖ "Should all of the above have come into play and resulted in the nurses simply seeking the insights of another nurse, double checking with the pharmacist, or heaven forbid, asking the doctor?"
 ➢ "Yup."

There are lots of drug references out there in electronic as well as print formats. We highly recommend you find one you like, have it somewhere easily accessible on your unit, <u>and use it</u>. It's especially important for high-risk, low-frequency medications like Vancomycin in a two-week-old child. Taking the time and expense to get it right is much better than dealing with the after effects of getting it wrong.

Moral of the story

If it doesn't look, sound, or seem right, it probably isn't. Whether it is a miscalculation, an errant decimal point, or simply an inappropriate order, your first priority is always the care and safety of your patient!

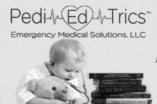

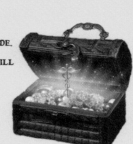

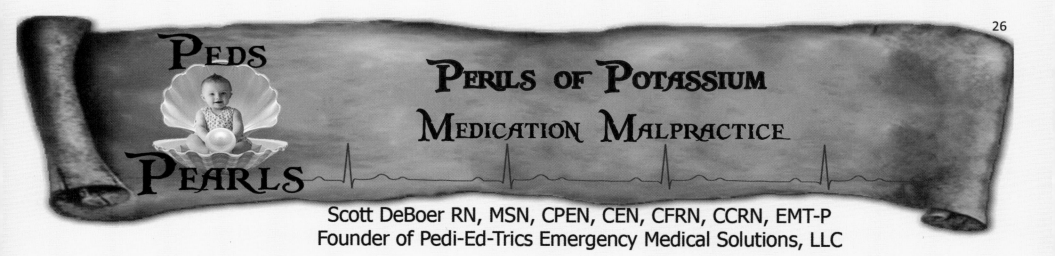

26

PERILS OF POTASSIUM
MEDICATION MALPRACTICE

Scott DeBoer RN, MSN, CPEN, CEN, CFRN, CCRN, EMT-P
Founder of Pedi-Ed-Trics Emergency Medical Solutions, LLC

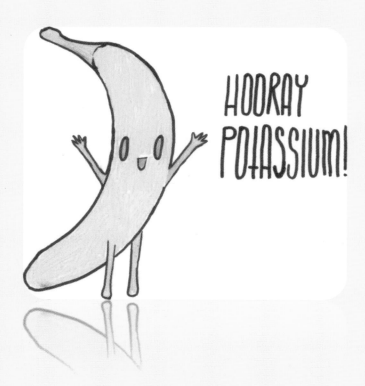

HOORAY POTASSIUM!

If it looks like way too big of a tube, it *probably is* way too big of a tube. If it seems like way too much fluid, it *probably is* way too much fluid. And if it sounds like way too big of a dose (even for big people), it *probably is* way too big of a dose (especially for a little one).

Scenario...

Several years ago, there was a tragic medical malpractice case that focused on a two-year-old little girl in an ICU after being intubated for respiratory failure. While in the unit, her potassium was low and an order was received for 120meq of oral potassium (via NG tube). While many nurses are comfortable and familiar with adult doses of oral potassium (K-lor, K-dur, etc.) of 20-40meq, it's a different story when the patient is a child. With children, we live in a weight-based world where everything is "something per kilo." This means that pediatric medication doses, in almost every case, must be calculated. Additionally, logic would suggest that pediatric doses will *probably be* smaller than adult doses.

In this case, the child didn't get all 120meq at one time, but instead, the nurse broke it down into three doses and gave 1/3 of the total dose (40meq) each hour for three hours. Shortly after the third dose, after receiving 120meq of oral potassium over just a few hours, the child went into cardiac arrest and was not able to be resuscitated.

In preparing for this case, the attorney for the child's family interviewed a nursing expert. Given the fact that the order was for 120meq of oral potassium and the child was only two-years old, some of the questions and answers discussed were along these lines:

❖ "Have you ever given potassium supplements to a two-year-old child in the ICU and if so, how often?"
➤ "Yup. All the time. It's usually given IV, but it's not uncommon to be given NG or PO."

❖ "Should the fact that this order was for 120meq have caught the attention of the nurses?"
➤ "Yup. Not only is it a big dose, but it's a <u>really</u> big dose. Big enough that most nurses have never given that much at one time to one patient, even a "big adult" patient."

❖ "Should all of the above have come together and resulted in the nurses simply seeking the insights of another nurse, double checking with the pharmacist, or verifying the dose with the fellow/attending?"
➤ "Yup."

Now this is where it gets interesting. To his or her credit, the nurse actually did check with the resident who confirmed the 120meq order. But should the nurse have "known better" and trusted his or her gut that this was <u>way too big</u> of a dose? Yes.

The medical examiner had multiple discussions with toxicology experts as to whether, in the absence of renal failure, is it possible to overdose a patient on oral potassium, and if so, could that potassium overdose be the cause of death? As expected, the answer was possibly yes. So, if you thought that it sounded like way too big of a dose for an adult and therefore, way too big of a dose for a little kid, you were absolutely correct.

Our Recommendation

There are lots of drug references in print and electronic formats out there. We highly recommend you find one you like, have it somewhere easily accessible, and use it (especially for high-risk medications like potassium). They are much cheaper than medication malpractice settlements!

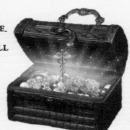

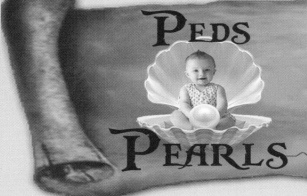

27

PEDS PEARLS

MG AND mL... MOVING AND PUSHING...
ADMINISTERING EPINEPHRINE AND AMIODARONE

Scott DeBoer RN, MSN, CPEN, CEN, CFRN, CCRN, EMT-P
Founder of Pedi-Ed-Trics Emergency Medical Solutions, LLC
Contributed by: Michael Rushing NRP, CCEMT-P, RN, BSN, CEN, CPEN, CFRN, CCRN-CMC

Pediatric Rarities and Stressful Situations

Pediatric full arrests are rare; some might say, "Incredibly rare." That's because pediatric ventricular fibrillation (VF) and pediatric ventricular tachycardia (VT) are similarly and incredibly rare. When those events do happen, they are incredibly stressful. And when faced with incredibly stressful situations, we do best when we need to remember less. So, it's fortunate for us that during the heat of battle, in the midst of incredible stress and confusion, we usually need to remember only two medications. The first is epi, epi, and more epi, and then only occasionally, amiodarone. Remembering that we commonly only push two meds for pediatric VF/VT, the next challenge is to find an easy way to remember the dosing for them. Well, today is your lucky day!

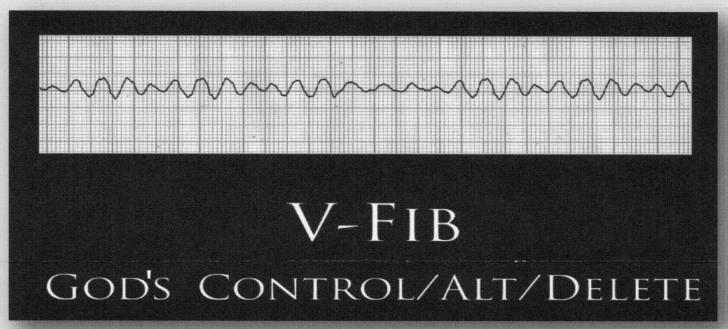

V-FIB
GOD'S CONTROL/ALT/DELETE

The **1:10,000** epinephrine that we push during a code (that familiar box of epi) only comes in one concentration - 1mg/10mL That makes epinephrine easy.

The amiodarone that we push during a code only comes in one concentration - 50mg/mL. That makes amiodarone easy.

The initial dose of epi is 0.01mg/kg and amiodarone is 5mg/kg (max 300mg). But that's way too many numbers and way too difficult to remember. There's got to be a better way! And there is because today really is your lucky day!

Decimals

Honestly, as far as medication administration goes during a pediatric code, all most of us care about is "How much should I push?" If you know (or can estimate) how much the kid weighs (in kg), simply move the decimal point in the weight one place to the left and that's your **dose of epi** in mL. If you know (or can estimate) how much the kid weighs (in kg), simply move the decimal point in the weight one place to the left and that's your **dose of amiodarone** in mL. How cool is that! Have you noticed a pattern here? Let's take a look at a few examples:

- A 50kg "funky heart kid" in V-fib should receive 5mL of epi and 5mL of amiodarone (50kg → 5mL)
- A 10kg kid who got into "Grandma's heart pills" in V-fib should receive 1mL of epi and 1mL of amiodarone (10kg → 1mL)
- A 3kg neonate in V-tach should receive 0.3mL of epi and 0.3mL of amiodarone. (3kg → 0.3mL). Watch out for these little ones – decimal points can be tricky and decimals really do make a difference!

Remember...

The above rule is only for how many milliliters to push, **NOT** for the milligrams you record. So, during a pediatric VF/VT arrest when you only push two drugs (epi and amio) and honestly only care about how much to push, there is a better way to remember the meds, and you just learned it! Just move the decimal point one time and that's your dose!

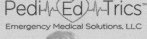

Pedi-Ed-Trics
Emergency Medical Solutions, LLC

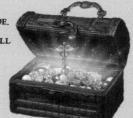

Info@PediEd.com 〰 1-888-280-PEDS (7337) 〰 PediEd.com

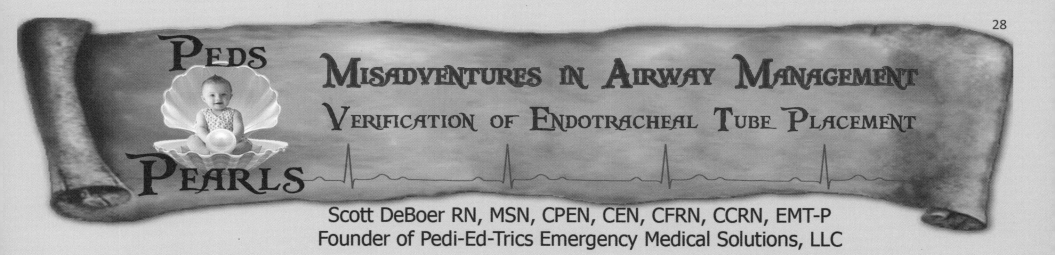

28

Misadventures in Airway Management
Verification of Endotracheal Tube Placement

Scott DeBoer RN, MSN, CPEN, CEN, CFRN, CCRN, EMT-P
Founder of Pedi-Ed-Trics Emergency Medical Solutions, LLC

> "An esophageal intubation is no sin, but there is great sin in not recognizing such a placement."

Where is the ETT?

When a patient is intubated, we want to confirm the proper placement of the endotracheal tube. We want to know **where** the ETT is located. Everyone knows that. And everyone knows that there is only one good answer to the question - **in the trachea**.

There is a second question that needs to be asked as well. **How** do we confirm the correct placement? The answer to the second question is not as simple as the first one.

There is (or at least there should be) an additional question which asks how correct placement is verified or confirmed over time. In other words, initially verifying correct placement doesn't necessarily ensure that the correct placement in the trachea is maintained.

Unfortunately, when we don't ask these questions initially, we find that they may be asked by attorneys during the course of medical malpractice cases. Nurses and physicians who have served as expert witnesses on these types of legal cases have been asked these questions all too often.

The key to avoiding these situations is knowing where your tube is at **all** times! This is an important consideration because "stuff" happens. Tubes that are correctly placed in the trachea can migrate into the esophagus, especially with children where the amount of "wiggle room" is very limited, but the wiggle potential is large.

So, if the answer to the first question is simple, how do you answer the follow-up questions? How do you verify and monitor the correct placement of your endotracheal tube? Chest X-ray… Breath sounds… Oxygen saturations… CO_2 color change devices… End-tidal CO_2 waveform measurements?

Answering the Questions

A chest X-ray is good for verifying initial placement and may even help identify adjustments that might be needed. But that chest x-ray is literally just a picture of a moment in time. It tells us nothing about where the tube was before, or more importantly, after the X-ray was taken.

Breath sounds are nice, but when it comes to little babies, you can put a tube almost anywhere and get air movement sounds almost everywhere. Oxygen saturation readings are also nice and we do like measurable signs, but such readings can lag behind the actual status of the airway. This means it can take a while for the sats to drop, even with a tube in the wrong place.

Colorimetric CO_2 detectors (color changing devices) like the Pedi-Cap (www.covidien.com) and MiniStat CO_2 (www.mercurymed.com) work well for several hours. If it turns gold, gold is good, and the tube is probably in the correct spot. If it turns purple and your patient turns purple, the tube is probably in the wrong spot. But these devices are generally qualitative rather than quantitative and have environmental and time-related limitations.

If available, end-tidal CO_2 measurement by way of <u>continuous</u> waveform capnography is the best answer. This not only gives you an actual CO_2 number, but also a continuous waveform to ensure that air is going in to and coming out of the right place. Just as continuous ECG monitoring allows you to watch the heart for any beat to beat changes, capnography allows you to monitor both respiration and ventilation. Transport nurse educator, Sean Smith, describes capnography as the "12-lead for the lungs" and anesthesiologist, Joan Spiegel, calls it "The most vital of vital signs!" If you have it, use it. If you don't have it, get it. It truly is invaluable for initial <u>and</u> ongoing verification of tube placement.

Proving the Answer

Should any question about the ETT placement arise, legal or otherwise, you should be able to rely on good documentation that would include:
- Presence of bilateral breath sounds initially and regularly throughout your care
- Regularly recorded vital signs (HR, BP, and O_2 sats)
- Documentation of end-tidal CO_2 readings as evidenced by recorded waveform capnography strips

It's as easy as that. If you document breath sounds, sats, and CO_2 readings throughout the episode and especially before and after <u>every</u> move <u>and</u> upon arrival to another unit, you will be able to state with confidence that you know where your tube was at all times. Taking just a few seconds to assess and document is much easier, much less time consuming, and ultimately much less expensive than participating in an airway "misadventure" malpractice legal action and/or settlement. And most importantly, it is the right thing to do for your patient! Every tube, every time. It's not enough for you to <u>know</u> where the tube is, you have to be able to <u>prove</u> where your tube is!

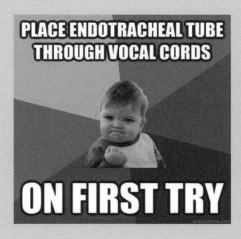

PLACE ENDOTRACHEAL TUBE THROUGH VOCAL CORDS

ON FIRST TRY

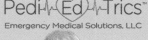
Pedi-Ed-Trics
Emergency Medical Solutions, LLC

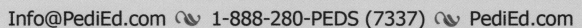

29

NEBS 101 - CLOSER IS BETTER
PEDIATRIC NEBULIZER TECHNIQUES

Scott DeBoer RN, MSN, CPEN, CEN, CFRN, CCRN, EMT-P
Founder of Pedi-Ed-Trics Emergency Medical Solutions, LLC
Insights from: Stu McVicar RRT, FP-C, CCEMT-P

Closer is Better

Whether it's wheezing, sneezing, or one of many other respiratory complaints, chances are pretty good that the child will be receiving a breathing treatment. Many of us are familiar with the acronym "HHN," which stands for Hand-Held Nebulizer and that's by far the most common method for administering a wide variety of respiratory medications. But when it comes to pediatric patients, while the "neb" concept remains constant, the "Hand-Held" part of the equation may present some interesting challenges, particularly with the youngest of our patients.

There is a little secret about how nebs work. First of all, "Yes, they really do work." But here's the little secret. They only work to the extent that the nebulized medication actually makes it to the bottom of the lungs. If the neb treatment is spraying those fine particulates into the room's air, the treatment will be less than optimally effective. So, the challenge we face is how to get the medication actually into the patient's lungs and not into their mouth, shirt, etc. Moral of the story - closer is better when it comes to nebs!

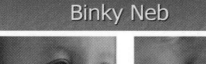

How Can I Help My Child Cooperate While Using the Nebulizer?

Challenge Part 1: All too often, the population needing the neb treatment has significant amounts of thick nasty snot. To get the best results out of ANY neb treatment, first make sure the patient's airway (mouth and nose) is as clear of secretions as it can be. Using a bulb syringe or a lubricated suction catheter works wonders! Keep in mind the nostrils go straight back, not straight up. As with head trauma patients, be careful with nasal suctioning. You want to suction out boogers, not brains!

Challenge Part 2: If you actually want the medication to reach the lungs, the neb treatment must enter the airway. In Zen terms, the medication must become one with the breathing. There are several paths to that level of enlightenment. If the child is old enough, wise enough, and strong enough to understand and follow instructions, the proverbial HHN device might work. And if all our patients were old enough, wise enough, and strong enough, we could end this pearl right here. But that's just not the case, so let's explore some alternatives.

Option 1: How about strapping or holding a neb mask to children's faces? Would that work? In some cases, "Yes." If they are sick enough to let you strap a mask to their face, they probably need to have a mask strapped to their face. However, if they need the treatment but are still well enough to rip the mask off their face, perhaps we can suggest some other options.

Option 2: What about the old-fashioned blow-by nebs? Do they work? The published research says, "No." But what about an alternative to the old-fashioned blow by delivery technique? Now that, as they say, is a horse (or a turtle, or a seal) of a different color. There are lots of cute nebulizer machines (seals, dogs, penguins, fire trucks, etc.) accompanied by cute masks (dragons, fish, turtles, elephants, etc.) that are available for both homes and hospitals, and they can make giving nebs to kids a lot less stressful.

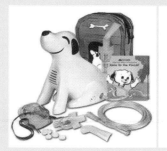
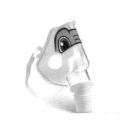

www.justnebulizers.com

Option 3: For children who won't keep a nebulizer mask on their face, there's the Pedi-Neb (aka Binky Neb). The concept is simple. The kid sucks on the binky and the neb is updrafted toward their nose. This works great because 1) Little ones like binkies, and 2) They like to breathe through their nose. However, many kids are very territorial about their binkies. And if it's not *their* binky, they don't want anything to do with it. This is easily overcome by dipping the binky in "Toot Sweet," "Sweet- Ease," etc. – some sort of sweet treat! The kid then happily sucks on the pacifier because of the sugar and gets the neb treatment at the same time. Just re-dip in the sugar solution PRN until the neb treatment is completed.

Binky Neb

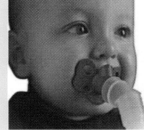
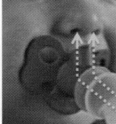

www.westmedinc.com

Remember…

When it comes to kids and nebs, whether it's with a cute mask or binky, to get the best results, get up close and personal!

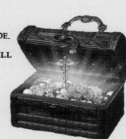

Info@PediEd.com ☏ 1-888-280-PEDS (7337) ☏ PediEd.com

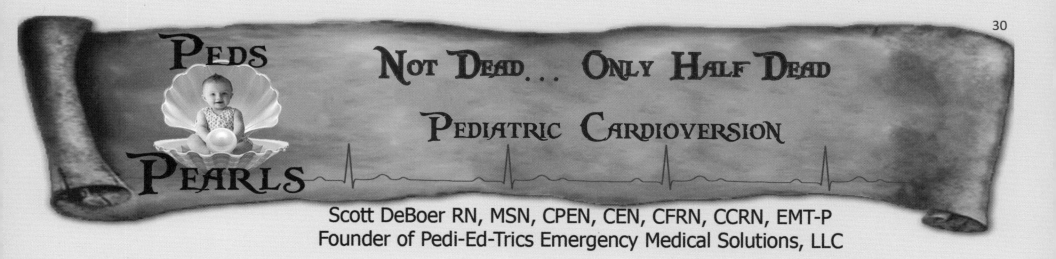

Scott DeBoer RN, MSN, CPEN, CEN, CFRN, CCRN, EMT-P
Founder of Pedi-Ed-Trics Emergency Medical Solutions, LLC

Defibrillators vs Drugs

We have many uses for electricity in the world of emergency medicine. We have lights, sirens, scopes, and monitors. We also have that machine called a defibrillator. Defibrillators, it should come as no surprise, are used for defibrillation. That's quite handy when your patient is in ventricular fibrillation (V-fib). Defibrillation begins with "D" and that's for dead people... not our favorite scenario.

And when we think of that particular machine and use of electricity, we should remember that "C," as in cardioversion, comes before "D" in the alphabet. So, what do you do if your patient is not in V-fib, but is in supraventricular tachycardia (SVT) with a rate that is clearly too fast? If they are conscious and able to say, "Please don't put those paddles on my chest," they probably don't need to have the paddles put on their chest. In that case, it would probably be very appropriate to consider the other "D" in our lexicon… drugs (adenosine, diltiazem, etc.). And even if your patient is unstable, but still at all conscious, drugs for sedation should seriously be considered before cardioversion. Shooting electricity through the chest really is not a pleasant experience!

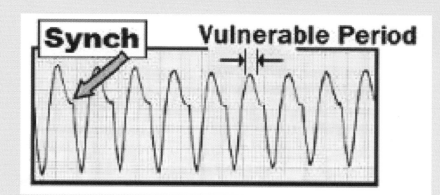

So, if your patient appears to be crashing right before your eyes, but is still alive with a pulse and a pressure, synchronized cardioversion is indicated. Cardioversion begins with a "C" and it's for patients who are "C"rashing. If your patient is not dead, but only "half-dead," the energy for cardioversion is half the defib dose (2j/kg) and that means 1j/kg. Yes, some peds cardiology centers who cardiovert kids on a regular basis use doses as low as 0.25-0.5j/kg, but in the ER, half the dead person dose is much easier to remember. In a very small child, it is distinctly possible that you won't be able to dial in the "exactly correct" dose for either defibrillation or cardioversion. You will often fall between numbers on the dial. If the dial choices are 15j and 20j, but you need 18j, go big (20j) or go home! Make sure you go over rather than under. It's like a reverse "Price is Right" game where you want to get closest, without going under, the formula amount.

"Sync"

Cardioversion is for the patient who still has a perfusing rhythm and when you want the electricity to be delivered at the right point of the cardiac cycle to avoid shocking the heart into V-fib. **It is crucial to remember to hit the "Sync" button** prior to each cardioversion attempt to ensure that cardioversion, not defibrillation, is done. Your patient has a pulse, rhythm, and a QRS complex; it's just REALLY fast. Defibrillating SVT can disrupt the QRS complexes and cause a full arrest. This would look really bad (and is so much more paperwork).

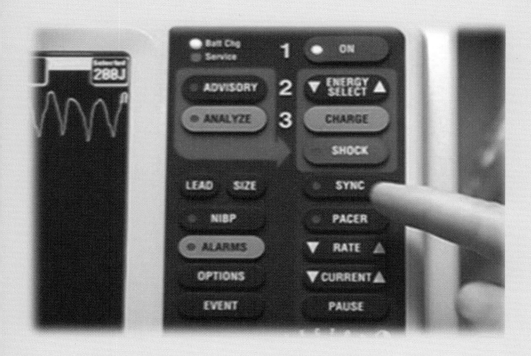

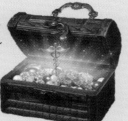

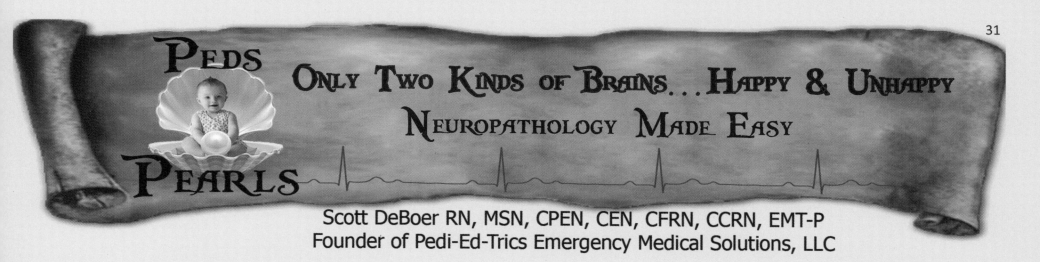

31

PEDS PEARLS

ONLY TWO KINDS OF BRAINS...HAPPY & UNHAPPY

NEUROPATHOLOGY MADE EASY

Scott DeBoer RN, MSN, CPEN, CEN, CFRN, CCRN, EMT-P
Founder of Pedi-Ed-Trics Emergency Medical Solutions, LLC

Brain Science?

Contrary to popular belief, understanding how the brain works is not complicated… it's not like brain surgery or anything. In fact, some people would say that it's as simple as 1,2,3. We all have just 1 brain, there are only 2 types of brains, and only 3 things that brains need.

Despite all the technology we carry around in our pockets (we often call them our backup brains), the brain we start with is the only brain we get. And there are really only two types of brains… happy brains and unhappy brains. So what is it that the brain needs to be happy? Only three things… blood, oxygen, and glucose.

1. **Blood:** Whether it be your heart, brain, or really anywhere in your body, if you don't have a regular supply of blood to the tissues, those tissues will become very unhappy and very unforgiving very quickly. (Consider the sequelae of strokes, heart attacks, etc.)

2. **Oxygen:** This goes hand in hand with blood. Getting oxygen to the brain is good and the brain stays happy. Not getting oxygen to the brain is bad.

3. **Glucose:** Glucose is virtually the sole fuel for the human brain, except during cases of prolonged starvation. The brain lacks fuel stores and hence, requires a continuous supply of glucose. Think about how you feel toward the end of an extended shift during which you haven't stopped to pee, let alone eat. Without that supply of "fuel," you become progressively more hungry and cranky (aka "hangry") as your brain is letting you know it is very unhappy.

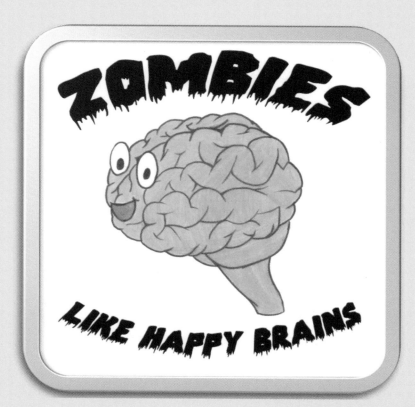

ZOMBIES LIKE HAPPY BRAINS

How this comes into play with pediatrics is simple. When called on to provide care to children, whether in an ambulance or the emergency department, and they are behaving in any way other than neurologically normal (or their baseline), do a fingerstick sugar and a pulse ox. Think about it. These are two of the three things that make your brain happy. And if it's not one of those two things, then you should be prepared for a trip to the CT machine. But, if the blood sugar or oxygen sat is low, you can quickly address that situation and your patient might not need the CT after all. How cool is that!

It's Simple...

Your brain only wants blood, oxygen, and glucose to be happy. So, check a pulse ox and always remember to check a blood sugar in your attempts to keep those brains happy and those kids warm, pink, and sweet. **It's as easy as 1, 2, 3!**

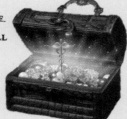

32

Peds Pearls

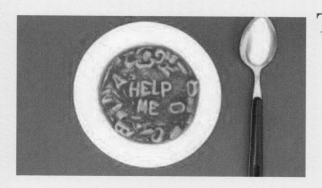

Passing TNCC and ENPC
Top Ten Test Taking Tips

Scott DeBoer RN, MSN, CPEN, CEN, CFRN, CCRN, EMT-P
Founder of Pedi-Ed-Trics Emergency Medical Solutions, LLC

Contributed by: Marlene Bokholdt RN, MSN; Vickie Dollhausen RN, MSN, CEN, CPEN, EMT-P; Michael R. Lovelace, RN, CEN,CFRN, CCEMTP, NREMTP, EMTP-T; Justin Milici MSN, RN, CEN, CPEN, CFRN, CCRN, and Michael Rushing NRP, RN, BSN, CEN, CPEN, CFRN, CCRN-CMC, CCEMT-P, BSN.

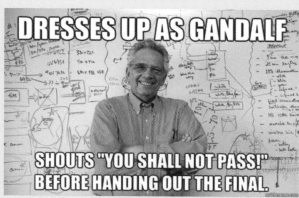

DRESSES UP AS GANDALF
SHOUTS "YOU SHALL NOT PASS!" BEFORE HANDING OUT THE FINAL.

Ahhh . . . alphabet soup emergency certification courses. What a truly fun way to spend a weekend! But seriously, they are a necessary part of our profession and actually do provide good information along with structured methods to guide assessments and patient management priorities. To aid in that learning process, some of our favorite and well-seasoned instructors have provided the following tips to help you pass certification courses such as the Emergency Nurses Association's Trauma Nursing Core Course (TNCC) or Emergency Nursing Pediatric Course (ENPC).

Take I:

Read the book. Read the whole book. The book is your best friend. Read the chapters WELL before coming to class, not the night before. The written test is based on the book, lectures, and skills stations. All of the answers are in the book somewhere. You just have to have read it and attend the full class to know the right answers.

Take II:

When doing a reassessment, many students forget what they should actually reassess besides the ABC's. One simple tip is to remember "3 P's and a V".

- **P**rimary Assessment
- **P**ain
- **P**roblem of the Patient
- **V**ital Signs

When the student is asked what to reassess, just remember the 3 P's and V. This covers all the injuries and ABC stuff.

The Top 10 Testing Tips:

1) Make sure you review the pre-test multiple times. Getting comfortable as to how questions are worded can be very helpful.

2) Understand and memorize the trauma or medical assessment steps you find in the back of the books.

3) Double starred items must be done and must be done in order. Single starred items must be done sometime. That bears repeating. The double starred items <u>cannot</u> be missed, must be done <u>in the correct order</u>, and must be completed before moving onto the next section. Notice that the double starred items are in the primary survey. A ** for the assessment item, and if abnormal, a ** for the intervention. For example, ** means that you must assess the airway for patency. If the airway is blocked with blood, snot, or other bodily fluids, there is a ** to suction. Single star items <u>must</u> be completed, but not necessarily in order. At the end of the scenario, the instructor will ask if there is "anything you would like to add or revise…" It doesn't necessarily mean that you have forgotten or messed up on anything. The instructors ask this of everyone. You can add (i.e. forgot to say and now remembered) the single star items*, but the primary assessment ** items MUST be stated prior to going onto the secondary assessment. It's like the point of no return at Niagara Falls. There is no going back!

4) Read the question carefully. If it is asking for an intervention, then pick an intervention. If it is asking for a priority, pick a priority answer. With priority questions, look for the ABC's unless there is life threatening blood loss.

5) Mnemonics, such as CIAMPEDS and PAT (Peds Assessment Triangle) for ENPC are your friends. Understand them, memorize them, live them, love them, and don't forget them. The A through I mnemonics are special cases because the "A through I" for TNCC are <u>quite different</u> from ENPC. And… DON'T forget to "I"nspect posterior surfaces. Thou must roll thy patients and examine their backs or thou hast only done 1/2 of the assessment and thou shalt surely be sorry!

6) If you get flustered during the testing scenarios, take a breath (and consider 5mg of Valium?), re-evaluate what you have done (primary survey, secondary survey, etc.), and then re-engage.

7) Remember TNCC and ENPC are "textbook" perfect situations. Your actual practice will likely be somewhat different. The scenarios are designed to be as realistic as possible, but an artificial situation will never be the same as real life. The instructors need you to work without your team and do things step-by-step to see what you know and can do. Even though real life involves a team and things are done simultaneously, this is a test and only a test; it is there to confirm that you have the skills and knowledge to be on the team.

8) Please ask questions. The question you have is probably the same question someone else has, but is too afraid to ask (just like in nursing school).

9) Slow down when in the scenarios and take your time on the written test. Unlike real life with crashing and dying patients, the scenarios and written tests are not timed tests.

10) When answering the test questions, go with your first choice and avoid changing your answer unless there is an overwhelmingly powerful reason to revise it.

Emergency certification courses are the entry level courses for many emergency departments. Just remember our top 10 tips as well as the "3 P's and a V" and you will have a greater chance of successfully passing TNCC and ENPC.

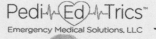

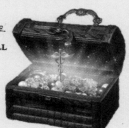

Info@PediEd.com ☏ 1-888-280-PEDS (7337) ☏ PediEd.com

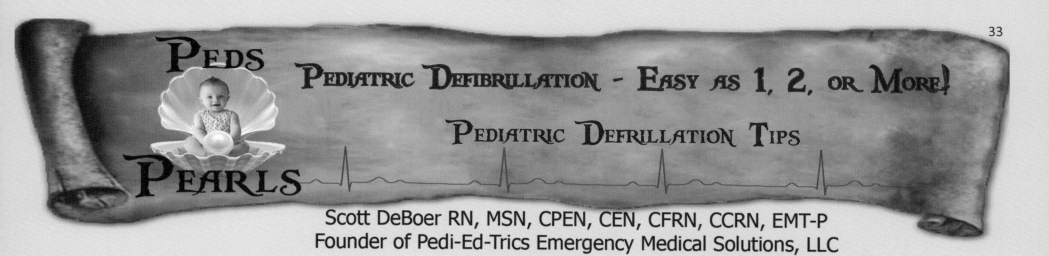

33

PEDS PEARLS

PEDIATRIC DEFIBRILLATION - EASY AS 1, 2, OR MORE!

PEDIATRIC DEFRILLATION TIPS

Scott DeBoer RN, MSN, CPEN, CEN, CFRN, CCRN, EMT-P
Founder of Pedi-Ed-Trics Emergency Medical Solutions, LLC

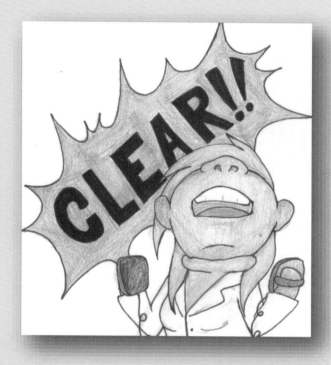

Number 1...
When dealing with the unlikely, but nonetheless horrible situation in which a child needs to be defibrillated, any tricks that help you to remember even the basic rules can help. So, first things first. Find the pads or paddles. But what size do you use once you find them? Pediatric pads or paddles (little ones) or regular size (big ones)? It's the *number 1* thing to remember and there is only 1 answer, so your clue is number 1. If the child is 1-year-old or younger, go for the smaller pads or paddles. Otherwise, go for the bigger ones if the child is bigger than 1!

Number 2...
The next challenge is the second, or *number 2* thing to remember, and that is the question of how much energy to use for the initial defib attempt. It's the second question, so your first clue is the number 2. But there is a second clue once you've selected the right size pads or paddles. That second clue is to pick up your paddles or pads and count them. There should be exactly 2. If there is anything but two, put them down, and ask someone else for help. Keeping in mind that everything in children is "something per kilo," the first defibrillation attempt should be at … you guessed it … 2j/kg. If the first attempt is unsuccessful, the second attempt is simply 2x2, or 4j/kg. This is true for subsequent attempts as well. Or is it?

More...
Is 4j/kg as high as we go? In the 2010 and 2015 PALS guidelines, there were little notations saying "… may consider up to 10j/kg." But many of us didn't give it a lot of thought because we were taught 2j/kg and then double to 4j/kg. It was easy to remember, and it got us the correct answers on the test. However, in a recently published pediatric defibrillation study (8-20% of pediatric cardiac arrests are first in V-fib after all), it was reported that 2j/kg did not work in a fair percentage of patients, and 4j/kg did not work in a fair percentage of patients, and that a much higher energy setting was needed to successfully convert pediatric VF.

To take that train of thought one step further… several years ago in Europe and Australia, they asked a very insightful question. If 2j/kg didn't work and then we are going to 4j/kg, why are we messing with 2j/kg? They routinely just start with 4j/kg and go up from there. The idea of starting high (4j/kg) and then going even higher (up to 10j/kg) is probably something you will be hearing about much more in the future.

Wait...
what if you have a little person and only big people paddles or pads? The American Heart Association currently recommends using the larger size as long as the pads or paddles don't overlap when placed on the child's chest. And you can slap one pad on the front and one on the back if needed. As discussed in another Peds Pearl about AEDs and kids, if all you have are the adult paddles or pads, go for it! The patient can't get any worse.

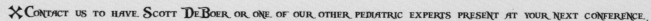

Info@PediEd.com ☏ 1-888-280-PEDS (7337) ☏ PediEd.com

34

PEDIATRIC PARKLAND
FLUID RESUSCITATION AND BURNS

Scott DeBoer RN, MSN, CPEN, CEN, CFRN, CCRN, EMT-P
Founder of Pedi-Ed-Trics Emergency Medical Solutions, LLC
Insights from: Annemarie O'Connor MSN, FNP-BC, APN/CNP

We all can understand why so many EMS or ER professionals consider kids to be such a challenge. And we certainly can understand why most consider kids that are burned an even bigger challenge. (Yes, that's the polite way of saying that they can scare the you-know-what out of us!) In conjunction with initial and ongoing fluid resuscitation, airway management and aggressive pain control are vital for the badly burned child's survival. Those other burn treatment priorities are covered in a separate Peds Pearl, so here are some thoughts specifically about fluid resuscitation for pediatric burn patients… A way to calculate <u>and hopefully remember</u> the infamous Parkland formula.

Things To Remember

Before we get into the actual calculations needed to figure out the formula, a few key reminders need to be given:

1) The formula is a guide, <u>not</u> the law! Some kids need more, some need less, but in the prehospital or ER arena, using the formula as a guide will get you in the right ballpark until instructed otherwise or until the patient arrives at a burn center.

2) The clock starts when the kid got burned, <u>not</u> when s/he arrives for your care. That's critically important. If a kid arrives several hours after the burn, you have some serious catching up to do.

3) Although the formula suggests lactated ringers (LR), some burn units prefer normal saline (NS). If you have a burn that is bad enough that you are actually calculating the formula, someone will probably be arranging immediate transfer to a burn unit. During the initial call to the receiving unit, simply ask which fluid (LR or NS) they prefer.

4) The formula is for fluid resuscitation. Little kids with big bad burns may be kept NPO and if that's the case, they will need maintenance fluids <u>in addition</u> to the resuscitation fluids. Maintenance fluids usually start with "D5" (like D5LR or D5NS). Again, this is in addition to the LR or NS resuscitation fluids.

5) The formula tells you more or less how much fluid the kid should receive in the first 24-hours post-burn. It is the total volume of fluid, but it is NOT divided equally over 24-hours. Your patient should get 1/2 of that big whomping amount in the first 8-hours as that's when the most fluid shifting and subsequent swelling takes place. The remaining fluid amount is given over the next 16-hours.

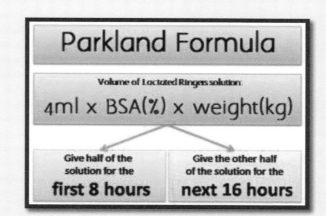

Parkland Formula

Volume of Lactated Ringers solution:

$$4mL \times BSA(\%) \times weight(kg)$$

Give half of the solution for the **first 8 hours**

Give the other half of the solution for the **next 16 hours**

The Parkland formula is **4mL x kg x % BSA** (body surface area) burned. The way that I've always remembered the 4mL x kg x BSA burn formula is to break it down like this:

4mL x

Look at your arms and legs and count them. How many are there? Four. Hopefully, they aren't burned, so you are doing better than the patient is.

Kg x

How much do they weigh in kg? With kids, pretty much everything we give is weight-based… something per kg. Another way to remember the weight component is simply that big kids get more fluids than little kids, so you'll be multiplying by a bigger number.

BSA burn

How much are they burned? Bad burns with a greater BSA burned get more fluids than not so bad burns. Like the bigger number with bigger kids, the bigger the burn area, the bigger the number you will be multiplying with to get total volume.

Multiply all three numbers together and that's how much fluid they get in the first 24-hours; <u>½ of that amount is to be infused in the first 8 hours</u>. Don't forget… this formula is just for burn fluid resuscitation. The child still needs IV maintenance fluids with dextrose as well.

Prehospital:

• **Short ETA** - Give a 20mL/kg bolus of LR or 0.9NS and the ER can figure out the rest.

• **Long ETA** - Figure out the formula and put the fluids on a pump if at all possible (it's much easier than counting drips).

ER:

• Figure out the formula and put the resuscitation fluids on a pump. Don't forget the maintenance fluids and put them on another pump.

Example: A 10kg child has 50% burns.
4mL x kg x BSA burns
- 4mL x 10kg x 50% = 2,000 mL over 24-hours.
- And ½ of that amount (1,000 mL) is to be given over the first 8-hours (125mL/hour x 8 hours).

Example: A 25kg child has 70% burns.
4mL x kg x BSA burns
- 4mL x 25kg x 70% = 7,000 mL over 24-hours.
- And ½ of that amount (3,500 mL) is to be given over the first 8-hours (437mL/hour x 8 hours).

Pediatric Parkland…
Remember:

1) Staying calm is good. So before you panic, remember you can always phone home (to the burn center) for help.

2) The Parkland formula is just for the burn fluids; the child still needs maintenance fluids too.

3) Sometimes, you just have to do the math!

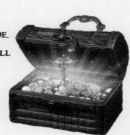

Info@PediEd.com ☏ 1-888-280-PEDS (7337) ☏ PediEd.com

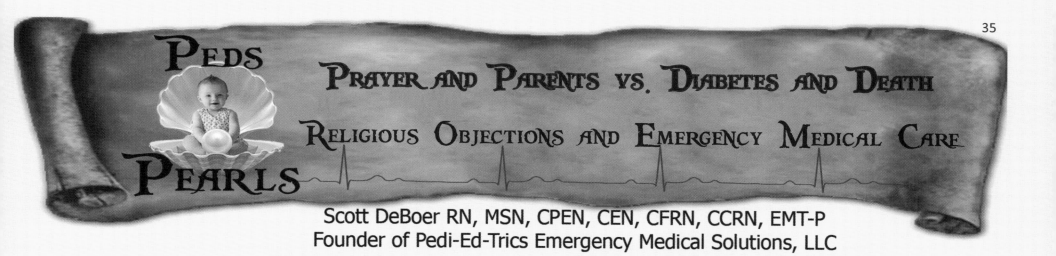

35

PEDS PEARLS

PRAYER AND PARENTS VS. DIABETES AND DEATH

RELIGIOUS OBJECTIONS AND EMERGENCY MEDICAL CARE

Scott DeBoer RN, MSN, CPEN, CEN, CFRN, CCRN, EMT-P
Founder of Pedi-Ed-Trics Emergency Medical Solutions, LLC
Contributed by: John R. Clark, JD, MBA, NRP, FP-C, CCP-C, CMTE

Imagine...

A 9-year-old girl who presents to the emergency department with a two-day history of abdominal pain and vomiting. The girl's mother advises the primary nurse that their family follows the "God Loves Glucose" religion. She further states that, consistent with the beliefs of her church, illness and injury can be cured through prayer, penitence and punishment; therefore, she began treating the girl through prayer. When her daughter was not feeling any better after three days, the mother became more concerned. At the urging of a family member who was not part of the church, Mom agreed to come to the hospital. Now, while we know that there is currently no Church of the Sacred Sugar or Gospel of Glucose, there certainly are groups whose religious beliefs can present challenges when faced with the need for modern medical treatment.

But in our imaginary scenario, as you develop a level of trust with the mother, she provides additional history that her daughter has been ill and increasingly lethargic for several weeks. Mom has noticed that the patient has lost a noticeable amount of weight despite "eating, drinking, and peeing all the time." Additionally, the young girl has been eating handfuls of sugary mints and candies in an attempt to cover up the unusual smell of her breath.

Having seen and heard all that you need to see and hear for now, a quick set of vital signs, coupled with a finger-stick glucose and capillary blood gas (or nasal cannula CO_2) confirm your suspicions of acute diabetic ketoacidosis (DKA). You share this information with the mother and quickly outline a plan of care that will help manage the diabetes and ultimately help save the child's life. Visibly upset, the mother now is having second thoughts about coming to the ER and wants to sign out against medical advice to take the child home. She expresses her belief that her daughter would best be treated by additional prayers, laying on of hands, and anointing with oils by church leaders.

Parents sometimes deny their children the benefits of modern medical care because of religious beliefs. Generally, when the physical or mental health of the child is at stake, the Supreme Court of the United States has long upheld the right of parents to make decisions for their children based on religious ground (the ethical belief of autonomy). But in cases of medical decisions affecting mortality or morbidity, the courts most often move to protect the minor child.

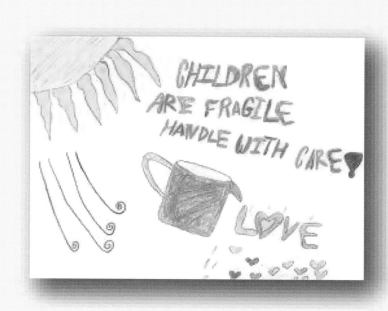

It's All About Balance

The courts must balance the rights of a parent against the interest and medical well-being of the child. What is very important here is how successful the treatment will be. If the proposed medical treatment has a good chance of success and the predicted outcome without treatment is death or long term disability, courts are more likely to intervene and overrule parental decisions. If the proposed medical treatment does not have a high likelihood of success, or the predicted outcome is not death or long term disability, courts frequently uphold the decision of the parents. The American Academy of Pediatrics issued a position statement in 2003 stating, "The AAP believes that all children deserve effective medical treatment that is likely to prevent substantial harm or suffering or death."

So, while your medical instincts scream loudly for you to do everything within your medical bag of tricks for every pediatric patient, we need to carefully weigh the needs of the child versus the rights of the parents.

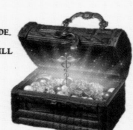

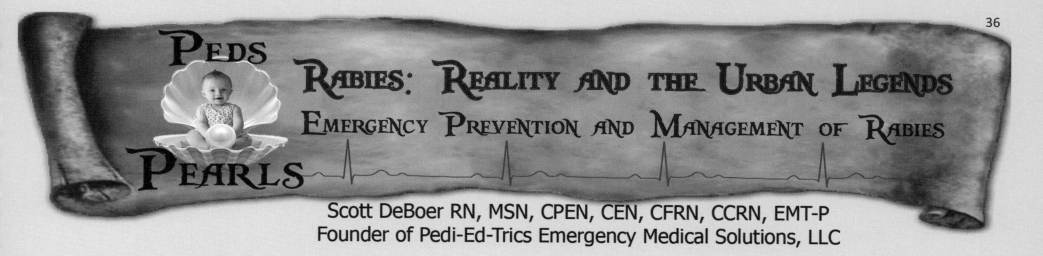

36

Rabies: Reality and the Urban Legends
Emergency Prevention and Management of Rabies

Scott DeBoer RN, MSN, CPEN, CEN, CFRN, CCRN, EMT-P
Founder of Pedi-Ed-Trics Emergency Medical Solutions, LLC

Many parents are convinced that if their child is bitten by a "strange" dog, immediate life-saving treatment is required. Why? Because they can remember hearing about the deadly menace of rabies, the huge scary needles, and the hundreds and hundreds of shots needed to stave off the grim reaper. We all remember those horror stories, but few of us have actual experience with rabies, and as such, we may have difficulty separating urban legend from reality.

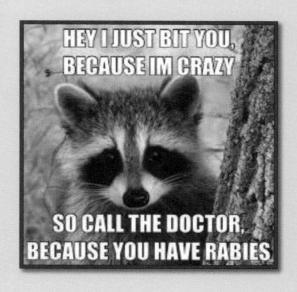

FINDS LUCKY RABBIT FOOT

GETS RABIES

Urban Legends

Urban legend holds that a confirmed diagnosis of rabies is a death sentence. This one is more truth than legend. Except in very rare cases, untreated rabies is fatal. That is, and should be, scarier than a diagnosis of ebola.

Urban legend also suggests that all pets (except our own) can or do carry rabies. This sounds like a gross over-generalization and indeed, it is. House pets, like dogs, cats, gerbils, parakeets, and goldfish are not at all likely to have rabies (especially the goldfish which aren't known for their tendency to bite or scratch). Other animals that might be called "pets," but aren't typically found indoors, are a different story; so, it is important to get the details about the animal bite circumstances. But again, pigs, llamas, and ferrets aren't likely carriers of rabies.

So, when should you worry about rabies? If you hear about a bite from a bat or a raccoon, that's when you should be concerned. Not all bats or raccoons carry rabies, but we do know that certain species of bats are the biggest carriers of rabies in the animal kingdom. Bites or scratches from a bat or raccoon mean the patient will most likely be receiving the full rabies series. The only exception to this would be if the family shows up with the offending animal and the animal is proven to be negative for rabies. Either way, the treatment starts immediately in the ER (or public health department) and the series continues until completed unless the rabies risk is definitively proven to be negative.

Another rabies-related urban legend is all about the hundreds of shots that are part of the treatment. This legend is perhaps exaggerated, but should not be totally dismissed. In summary, the patient potentially exposed to rabies gets rabies immune globulin injected into the bite itself (and other body areas as well depending on the child's weight), but that's not all. No, no! That's just for starters! They also get introduced to the rabies vaccine on days 1, 3, 7, and 14.

That's not the whole story... Giving those rabies shots is different from other injections we normally administer. That fact may contribute to the ferocity of the urban legends. Normally, if we have to give children an intramuscular injection, we load everything possible into the same syringe so they only receive one shot. But can you do that with rabies? Regrettably, no. It has to be two shots with two needles in at least two different sites.

Long Live the Legend

Now that we know how rabies is contracted and how it is treated, how do we prevent rabies? A simple answer is to stop children from playing with animals they shouldn't be playing with. But is that really possible? Do children follow rules just because an adult says to do so? We all know the answer to that. So, to increase the odds of adherence and decrease the risk of rabies, maybe it isn't such a bad idea to maintain some of the urban legends surrounding rabies. After all, there is that old saying about an ounce of prevention being worth a pound of cure. Kids don't need to be afraid of tame house pets, but maybe they can be influenced to avoid being in close proximity of "wild" animals, especially bats and raccoons. If we don't dismiss the cure (treatment) part of the urban legend, aka the part about the huge scary needles and hundreds and hundreds of shots, maybe it will help the prevention thing. The story about the kid down the block who got a hundred and nineteen shots in his stomach with a needle the size of a screwdriver might be just the incentive that is needed. Long live the legend!

Rabies exposure is relatively easily prevented and painfully treated, but if not treated, it's just about never cured.

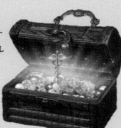

HEY I JUST BIT YOU, BECAUSE IM CRAZY

SO CALL THE DOCTOR, BECAUSE YOU HAVE RABIES

Info@PediEd.com 📞 1-888-280-PEDS (7337) 📞 PediEd.com

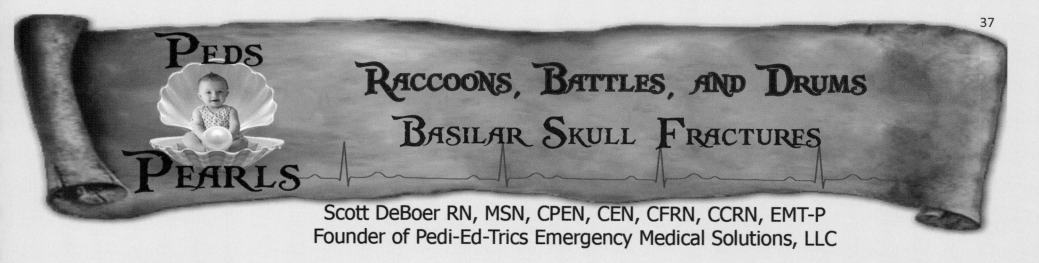

37

PEDS PEARLS

RACCOONS, BATTLES, AND DRUMS
BASILAR SKULL FRACTURES

Scott DeBoer RN, MSN, CPEN, CEN, CFRN, CCRN, EMT-P
Founder of Pedi-Ed-Trics Emergency Medical Solutions, LLC

Scenario…

As a result of a high-speed motor vehicle crash, a two-year-old is in the ER after flying into the automobile windshield. He is unresponsive, seizing, and is noted to have bruising around his eyes, bruising behind his ear, and clear fluid dripping from his nose. What are these findings called and, more importantly, what do they mean?

In school, many of us were taught about several assessment findings that were commonly associated with **basilar skull fractures** (fractures of the base of the skull). Those findings included **periorbital ecchymosis** (raccoon eyes), **mastoid ecchymosis** (bruising behind the ears, also known as Battle's sign), and **hemotympanum** (bleeding behind the ear drum). Basilar skull fractures are one of the most serious type of skull fractures and may also involve a tear of the dura resulting in leaking or dripping cerebrospinal fluid from the ears or nose.

Raccoon eyes: This is periorbital bruising involving one or both eyes and is a result of blood tracking down from the fracture site into the soft tissue around the eyes. Just picture a cute raccoon at the zoo (versus those going through your garbage) and that's raccoon eyes.

Battle's sign: This is bruising behind one or both ears (the mastoid process) and is a result of blood tracking there from a skull fracture often at the middle cranial fossa. This specific type of bruising is not from damage directly to the mastoid process. Named after Dr. Battle who first identified this type of ecchymosis, it's easy to picture medieval soldiers who got hit on the side of the head with a big 'ol mace. As they got their heads seriously messed up in battle, that's Battle's sign.

Hemotympanum: This is bruising behind the ear drum. Picture otitis media (ear infection), but this time, it's blood dripping into the space from the skull fracture, not pus.

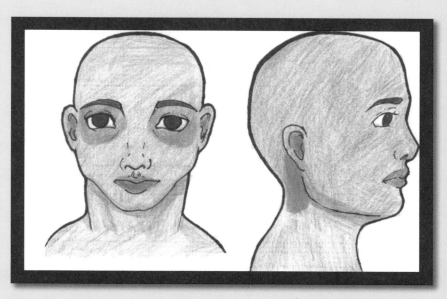

When it comes to bruising around the eyes or behind the ears, it's important to remember a few things:

1) Yes, this does happen with basilar skull fractures, but not all the time.

2) Yes, it does happen, but it isn't commonly found on the scene by EMS and isn't always visible in the ER. That's important. Like other bruises, it takes time to actually develop into a visible bruise. This means that if you follow up on a kid the next day in the Pediatric ICU and they have horrible bruising around their eyes, you can tell the PICU nurse, "I swear those weren't there yesterday when I took care of the kid." True. You didn't miss it. They just weren't there yet!

3) Depending on the age of the child and the reported mechanism of injury, always consider non-accidental trauma, aka a polite way of describing child abuse.

Moral of the story

After trauma, if you see bruising around the eyes, bruising behind the ear, or clear fluid dripping out of anywhere on the head, it's a basilar skull fracture until proven otherwise!

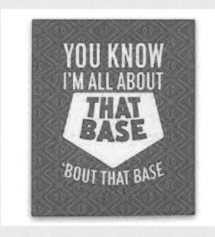

Info@PediEd.com ❧ 1-888-280-PEDS (7337) ❧ PediEd.com

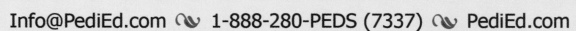

38

PEDS PEARLS

SANDBAGS, SUFFERING, EPIDURALS, AND EVERY BREATH YOU TAKE

FLAIL CHESTS

Scott DeBoer RN, MSN, CPEN, CEN, CFRN, CCRN, EMT-P
Founder of Pedi-Ed-Trics Emergency Medical Solutions, LLC

Breaking one rib is bad. Breaking two ribs is worse. Breaking at least two ribs in at least two places is even worse. And that's the classic definition of flail chest. Let's take a look at how we recognize it and how we treat it.

Evaluation (mechanism of injury):
Even before we can start X-rays, we can use our common sense and training to consider the history or story of the incident, i.e., a motor vehicle collision where an unbelted teenager (moveable object) hits a steering wheel (immovable object) at a high rate of speed; that's a pretty bad incident. Or, imagine a two-year old child who falls out of a fourth-story window; that's certainly a serious situation as well. Both certainly fit the "significant mechanism of injury" category and deserve diagnostic imaging.

Evaluation (physical exam):
If the kid looks crummy, can't breathe worth a darn, and has sats of 80% on room air, that's easy. There's a chest problem. But sometimes looks can be deceiving. And simply asking a kid if his chest hurts may not give you a truthful answer. Kids in pain sometimes deny it because if they say it hurts, that means they get a shot. So a trick that a peds ER doc shared with me works really well. Play a game where you slowly count their ribs. And as you count, push against the ribs. 1, 2, 3, 4, ouch! Ouch (or wincing or withdrawing) is the magic signal that tells you the likely location of an injury. Don't be surprised if that's the broken one.

And what about that paradoxical motion that we remember from school? That's where one side or section of the chest goes up and the other goes down; it's kind of like a see-saw. That is a good sign that something clearly is not right, but it <u>only</u> occurs in patients who are breathing spontaneously. That's important to remember as intubated patients won't show the see-saw or paradoxical motion.

Last, but not least, the increased work of breathing (without signs of airway problems like asthma, allergies, or obstructions) is also a good clue. Interestingly enough, the severity of the work of breathing is not related so much to the number of broken ribs, but to the underlying lung damage (pulmonary contusion, pneumothorax, etc.) beneath the broken ribs.

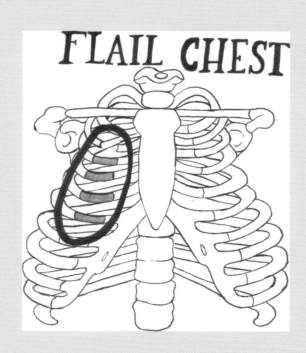

Evaluation (radiology):
Plain old X-rays (AP chest, rib films, etc.) can provide quick and easy identification of broken ribs. But it can be easy to miss a fracture. In many cases, if there's reason (back to mechanism and physical exam) to think about scanning the kid's chest for another reason (aortic injury), then radiology will find the fractures as well (bonus). On the adult side, some centers are having nice results using ultrasound to identify broken ribs without the need for radiation exposure.

Management (past and pulmonary):
In the not so distant past, the standard of care for flail chests involved intubation and mechanical ventilation with PEEP to stabilize the flail "from the inside out." But prior to PEEP, some experienced practitioners remember other recommended "remedies" including sandbag stabilization. But think about telling your patient, "I realize you have several crunchy broken ribs and are having a really hard time breathing. Let me put a 12# (5kg) sandbag on your chest. I'm sure that will help your ability to breathe immensely!" Understandably, that treatment plan is not as popular as it once was.

Management (pain):
For several years, caring for flail chests has really revolved around pain management. The ribs will heal with time, but as the song goes, "Every breath you take, every move you make…," they hurt! Pulmonary contusions, aka lung bruises, are commonly found under the broken ribs, and with time and respiratory care, they too will heal. But until the lung tissue and ribs heal, they hurt!

So, you can give your patient a whole lot of morphine and now they are pain free, but what do they forget to do? Breathe. Not an ideal situation. So, what are our other options for pain relief?

- **Intercostal nerve blocks**: These involve anesthesia injecting both sides of the broken ribs with long-acting local anesthetics every 12-hours. It works well, but involves multiple painful shots and anesthesia availability to regularly perform the procedure.

- **Epidurals:** Just like a C-section, but they thread it a little higher. When properly placed, they do a really nice job with pain relief and help get the patient off the vent sooner or keep them off the vent altogether.

- **Patient controlled analgesia (PCA):** Just like with post-op or sickle cell patients, PCA pumps paired with nasal cannula end-tidal CO_2 monitoring work really well to ward off pain while keeping the patient monitored and breathing on their own.

- **Surgery**: Recently, there have been several research studies published (primarily adult focused) detailing very positive pulmonary and pain relief experiences with early surgical fixation of the broken ribs. As with ultrasound diagnosis of broken ribs, this started with adults, but will very possibly extend into pediatrics in the near future.

Bottom Line

Kids have very flexible ribs and it takes a lot to break their ribs. Using your physical assessment skills and with the help of diagnostic imaging, you'll be able to tell if the trauma was sufficient to break a rib. And if they break not only one, but two or more ribs in two or more places, that's a flail chest. Once you know what you're dealing with, remember that as you manage their pain, you can manage the flail!

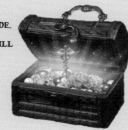

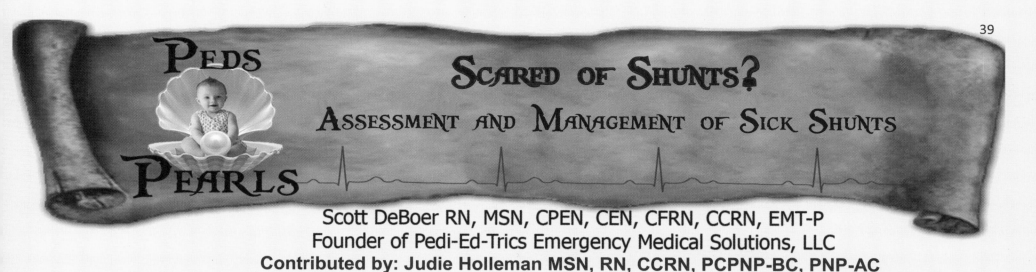

39

SCARED OF SHUNTS?
ASSESSMENT AND MANAGEMENT OF SICK SHUNTS

Scott DeBoer RN, MSN, CPEN, CEN, CFRN, CCRN, EMT-P
Founder of Pedi-Ed-Trics Emergency Medical Solutions, LLC
Contributed by: Judie Holleman MSN, RN, CCRN, PCPNP-BC, PNP-AC

The transfer center calls to inform you about an incoming patient transport with a possible V-P shunt malfunction. So, before the patient arrives, it's time to try to figure out what might be going on. Neurosurgical issues might seem complicated, so let's break them down into manageable pieces.

First of all, we should remember that what is actually being shunted is **Cerebral Spinal Fluid (CSF)**. Circulation of CSF is dependent on properly functioning ventricles in the brain, similar to how blood circulation is dependent on properly functioning ventricles (of the heart). If there is a problem with the brain ventricles, CSF accumulates in and around the brain and can result in a very dangerous pressure situation. When that happens, relief may be required in the form of a drainage conduit, typically from the ventricles of the brain to the peritoneal cavity (the belly), aka the creation of a ventriculo-peritoneal (VP) shunt. Unfortunately, those V-P shunts may shift, migrate, be outgrown, or just plain fail for some reason or another. And that situation, as you have probably guessed, is known as a V-P shunt malfunction.

The shunt that should be diverting the CSF is no longer diverting the CSF. So, the fluid either accumulates in the head or accumulates in the abdomen. Fluid collecting in either place doesn't allow the CSF to drain like it should and ultimately, the CSF will build up in the brain!

One thing to remember about kids with shunts is that if they have had a shunt malfunction before, they will typically (but not always) present with the same symptoms of increased intracranial pressure (ICP). Part of the initial assessment is to simply ask the parent/guardian if the present symptoms are similar to a previous shunt malfunction. Then, we should ask how long the child has been sick like this. Shunt malfunctions are not commonly a sudden onset event with rapid decompensation (with nasty symptoms like crashing, burning, and herniating in front of your eyes). It can get that bad, however, if the shunt has been malfunctioning for days or possibly even weeks. If the current symptoms include an elevated temperature or white blood cell count, keep in the mind the very likely possibility of an accompanying infection!

Symptoms:
If the child is complaining of a headache, be sure to check for the presence of an upgaze (ability to look up). Even kids who have lower baseline neurologic function will tend to follow a toy or an object and this is an easy way to test their upgaze. The lack of upgaze is an early subtle sign of acutely increasing ICP; the inability to control upgaze is a sign of cranial nerves III and IV dysfunction; the inability to maintain a midline pupil position, like sunset eyes, is a late, not so subtle sign. The ability to look up is a good sign. If you can only look up, that's a bad sign.

Ventriculoperitoneal (VP) Shunt

Entry to Cranium

Enlarged Left Ventricle

Valve (Behind Ear)

Underneath Skin

Extra Tubing in Peritoneal Cavity for Growth

Other symptoms of progressively increasing ICP from shunt issues are the same as with increased ICP from trauma. The cascade of symptoms might include headache, to headache and sleepy, to sleepy headache with vomiting, to decreasing responsiveness with sleepy vomiting headache, to unresponsive vomiting headache with posturing, to a blown pupil, to Cushing's Triad with sky high blood pressure, bradycardia, and irregular breathing, and finally central herniation and death.

Diagnostics:
If the symptoms are suggestive of a V-P shunt malfunction, diagnostic imaging should be expected.

One of the radiographic studies likely to be ordered is a shunt series. The shunt series includes plain X-rays of the shunt locations (head, neck, chest, and abdomen). The shunt series will show the entire length of the shunt tubing. If there is a disconnection or interruption of the tubing continuity, it will be in one of three places where tubing connects to tubing. Those places are:

1) In the head, where the ventricular catheter exits the skull and attaches to the reservoir.
2) Above or below where the reservoir tubing attaches to the valve (on the top of one side of the head).
3) Where the valve tubing connects to the tubing headed to the abdomen (in the neck or chest).

Many disconnections are easy to see on the X-ray often accompanied with comments like, "Wow, that tube in the neck is nowhere near the other piece of tubing coiled in the abdomen." Some are more subtle and may take an experienced radiologist or neurosurgery professional to find.

Other imaging studies used to rule in/out a shunt malfunction are a plain head CT or a rapid MRI to assess the ventricles. If the ventricles are way too big, it is likely the shunt is not working and CSF is accumulating. If that is the case, as you can imagine, the shunt probably needs to be revised.

Outcomes:
Remember that the severe signs (Cushing's) are late and truly ominous signs of impending doom for the child. In these cases, immediate drainage (tapping the shunt) and subsequent surgical revision or placing an External Ventricular Drain (EVD) is indicated to decrease the pressure on the brain and brain stem. But the vast majority of shunt malfunction kids are minimally to moderately symptomatic and very stable. It's not uncommon for them to be scheduled for surgery the next day unless they present during "regular working hours" and can be fitted into the OR schedule. Shunts can be scary, but if the parents or you catch the subtle signs before there is a major malfunction, the chance of a really good outcome is really good!

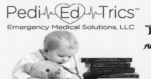

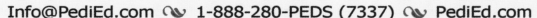

40

PEDS PEARLS

SHAKEN, NOT STIRRED

SHAKEN BABY SYNDROME

Scott DeBoer RN, MSN, CPEN, CEN, CFRN, CCRN, EMT-P
Founder of Pedi-Ed-Trics Emergency Medical Solutions, LLC

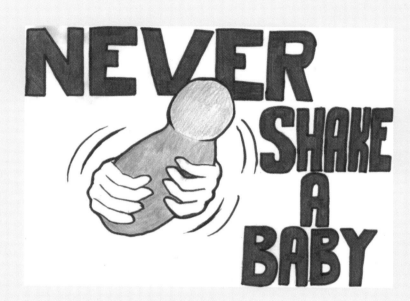

According to many nurses and medics, the only thing worse than a sick kid is a really sick kid. And the only thing worse than a really sick kid is an abused kid. Any parent, if they are honest, understands how difficult it can be when a new element is introduced to an already complex environment. That difficulty increases exponentially when the newly added factor is a helpless and very demanding baby. But when it changes from recognizing the difficulty to actually taking out that frustration on a child, that's when the line is crossed. And crossing that line, in all too many cases, results in Shaken Baby Syndrome.

As an introductory reference point:

- Roller coasters produce 3-4G of force

- Fighter pilots experience 6G of force

- <u>Shaking</u> a baby causes up to 9.3G of force

- If a child's head is struck against a solid object, forces increase <u>50-fold</u> to 428G!

So, when do we think about Shaken Baby Syndrome? In most cases, two criteria come into play:

1) **Age** – Babies up to one year, especially those 2 – 4 months of age, are at highest risk. Along with age are developmental milestones which need to be considered when evaluating the history and the reported mechanism of injury.

2) **History** – If the history keeps changing or doesn't fit the nature of injury, that's a big red flag.

If Shaken Baby Syndrome is suspected, we should expect the medical examination to include two specific things – a head CT and a retinal evaluation.

CT scan findings – A subdural bleed, or even worse, bilateral subdural bleeds (or other intracranial bleeds) in the presence of a story that doesn't fit is a significant factor in the diagnosis of Shaken Baby Syndrome.

Retinal hemorrhages – Up to 90% of kids diagnosed with Shaken Baby Syndrome are found by ophthalmologists to have retinal hemorrhages; that's one heck of a significant finding. It's important for ER physicians/mid-levels to look at the eyes, but if Shaken Baby Syndrome is being considered, having an ophthalmologist take a peek is crucial. An ER doc never wants to be the sole person who documented retinal hemorrhages, especially if they don't often see this finding. Obtaining an ophthalmology evaluation is crucial in arriving at a correct diagnosis as other things besides shaking can cause retinal hemorrhages. In addition, other findings can look like retinal hemorrhages to non-ophthalmologists and those other findings may not be associated with Shaken Baby Syndrome.

With few exceptions, it all adds up like this:

    A small infant

  + A history that doesn't fit the nature of the injury or is inconsistent

  + Subdural hematomas (or other intracranial bleeds) on CT scan

  + Retinal hemorrhages

  = Shaken Baby Syndrome

Info@PediEd.com ☏ 1-888-280-PEDS (7337) ☏ PediEd.com

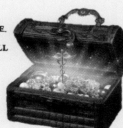

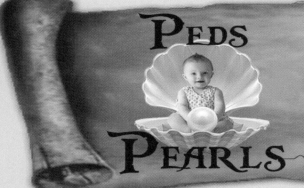

41

SUFFERING, SUFFOCATING, AND STROKING
SICKLE CELL EMERGENCIES

Scott DeBoer RN, MSN, CPEN, CEN, CFRN, CCRN, EMT-P
Founder of Pedi-Ed-Trics Emergency Medical Solutions, LLC

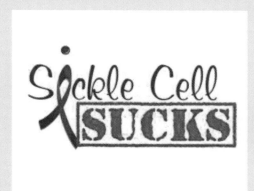

"Frequent Fliers"... In the EMS or ER world, that term evokes images of patients seeking seemingly constant attention for physiological or psychological conditions. All too often, those images are of a negative nature. Nevertheless, we have an obligation to provide appropriate medical care to all, regardless of circumstance. Patients living with sickle cell disease may be among those we see as "frequent fliers" and those individuals can be challenging for us. However, the more we know, the better prepared we are. So, with that in mind, let's explore some important factors regarding the nature and treatment of sickle cell disease.

Suffering: One of the most common reasons that we see patients with sickle cell disease is for management of a vaso-occlusive crisis, also known as a "pain crisis." When the abnormal sickled (crescent shaped) RBCs become stuck in the smaller blood vessels and capillaries, it can cause blockages and lead to tissue ischemia which results in severe pain. The pain crisis can come on quite suddenly and some of the more common triggers include dehydration and changes in body temperature. The severe pain can manifest itself in any part of the body and can be severe enough to send the patient (and parents) to the hospital seeking pain relief! Fortunately, after age 10, the rates of painful crises <u>decrease</u>, but the rates of complications <u>increase</u>!

Here are some of factors regarding treatment for those suffering from pain related to sickle cell disease:

- **Oxygen**: If they ask for oxygen, feel free to provide it. If they are short of breath, this treatment seems self-explanatory. What makes the treatment for these patients different is the fact that some experts recommend supplemental oxygen if the oxygen sats are less than 95% (not <90%).

- **Fluids**: If the patients are not dehydrated and able to tolerate PO fluids, PO fluids work just fine. If they are dehydrated or in need of IV fluids for other reasons (antibiotics, analgesia), certainly an IV or IO is appropriate. In some facilities, another option is the administration of subcutaneous (SQ) fluids and medications including saline, morphine, and Dilaudid (hydromorphone). For patients whose veins tend to be almost non-existent on a good day, SQ (or even elective intraosseous with local anesthesia) infusions can come to the rescue!

- **Pain Medication**: Experienced practitioners remember giving Demerol, Demerol, and more Demerol. Recently, however, the American Academy of Pediatrics has developed a formal position statement on the treatment of sickle cell pain. Essentially, it says 1) Demerol (meperidine) is not so good, 2) There are much better pain meds out there, and 3) If a sickle cell patient has never received Demerol, it would be better to avoid it altogether, and provide alternative medications instead. The many problems with Demerol include 1) Outside of anesthesia, very few providers give enough Demerol, 2) If you do give enough Demerol, patients tend to barf all over the place, and 3) The metabolites from boatloads of Demerol in kids can induce nasty seizures. Given that background, it is easy to understand the evolving role of Benadryl (diphenhydramine), NSAIDS (Ibuprofen, Toradol [ketorolac], etc.) and either oral, IV push, or PCA pump morphine or Dilaudid.

- **Protocols:** In terms of sickle cell pain crisis treatment, one of the best things that has come about recently is the development of protocols seen in many ERs. What that means is that when a patient presents in a pain crisis, the "clock" starts immediately and treatments begin. Then, after a specified amount of time, if the patient is still in pain, additional treatments/medications are given. Reassessments and additional orders continue as part of a predetermined treatment plan as time goes on. As the protocol is followed, there is a point at which the decision is made as to admit or discharge home. It makes our job a whole lot easier and provides consistent patient care regardless of the attending provider. Protocols also tend to eliminate the "doctor shopping" that some "frequent fliers" exhibit.

- **Addiction:** Addiction potential can be a real concern for some providers, but when it comes to the management of sickle cell pain crises, one wise pediatric emergency physician suggested the following:

"If I go to work every day and I have 100 patients in pain and if 99 of them are truly in pain and one is addicted, that means I have a 99% chance of making people feel better. If I make 99 children feel better, and feed one person's addiction, I'm OK with those odds."

Suffocating: The number one reason patients with sickle cell disease die is an acute or "clogged up" chest. If the sickle cell disease patient presents with chest pain, shortness of breath, and hypoxia, we have a seriously different situation. If a chest X-ray reveals a big infiltrate, it is probably either pneumonia or an acute chest. So in the ER, we simply treat them for both. The patient gets antibiotics, pain meds, and oxygen, and then once admitted, and with more time and extensive testing, it can be determined which of the two conditions are at play.

Stroking: The triad of really bad things that can come with sickle cell disease includes pain crises, acute or clogged up chest, and in the worst case, sickle cell stroke. As you can imagine, sickle cell stroke is a true emergency and often requires an exchange transfusion. The younger the kid is when experiencing their first sickle cell stroke, the higher the chance is of having another one. Additionally, if a young child's disease is bad enough to actually cause a stroke, then incredibly close follow-up is needed to prevent the devastating sequelae of more sickle cell strokes.

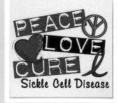

The overwhelming majority of pediatric sicklers hurt. They are praying you will treat their suffering while the parents and the peds ICU pray they don't suffocate or stroke!

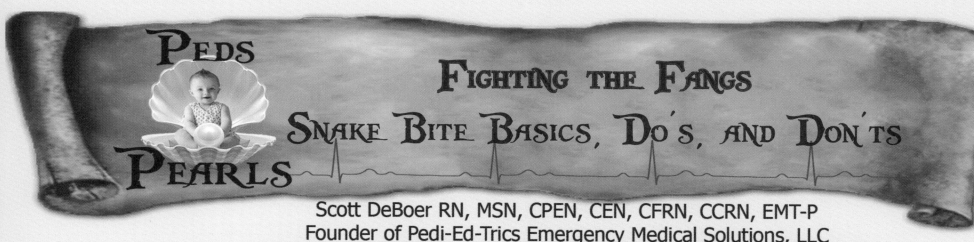

42

FIGHTING THE FANGS
SNAKE BITE BASICS, DO'S, AND DON'TS

Scott DeBoer RN, MSN, CPEN, CEN, CFRN, CCRN, EMT-P
Founder of Pedi-Ed-Trics Emergency Medical Solutions, LLC
Insights from: Michael Rushing NRP, RN, BSN, CFRN, CEN, CPEN, CCRN-CMC
& Steven Rogge RN, BSN, CEN, CCRN, CFRN, FAWM

Superman had his Kryptonite, Dracula had his sunlight, and Indiana Jones had his snakes. While most of us have little to fear about the first two, snakes (and their bites) can present a very real danger to us as possible victims and very real challenges to us as emergency medicine providers.

Important Do's and Don'ts regarding snake bites:

Do: Call poison control. They provide invaluable guidance for snake bites as well as potentially toxic ingestions.

Do: Definitely monitor your patient for signs of airway and cardiovascular compromise.

Do: Make sure your patient has at least one large bore IV and consider providing supplemental oxygen.

Do: With poison control guidance, consider the early administration of Crotalidae Polyvalent Immune Fab (CroFab). Since this antivenin is only for certain types of snakes, call poison control first!

Do: If administering CroFab, start the infusion slowly and then increase the rate from there. Watch for allergic reactions. While urticaria (itchy rash) is the most commonly reported side effect, it is not nearly as common as with the earlier types of antivenin. Patients receiving CroFab must be closely monitored for anaphylactic reactions, especially for those patients with a known allergy to papaya. (Papain, a papaya extract, is used in the production of CroFab.)

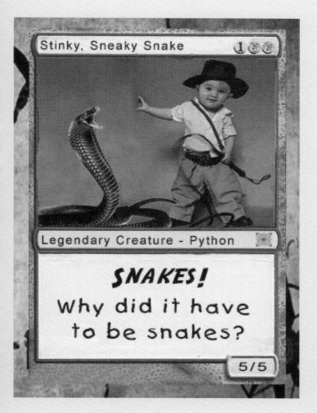

Stinky, Sneaky Snake 1🌑🌑

Legendary Creature - Python

SNAKES!
Why did it have to be snakes?

5/5

Do: Give the patient lots of IV pain meds as snake bites hurt really, really bad.

Do: If the patient or family has a picture of the snake on their phone, save it. Poison control may ask you to e-mail it to them for additional insights as to the type of snake that you are dealing with.

Do: Swirl the CroFab.
Don't: Shake the CroFab. If you shake it, you will just create a lot of foam and delay the administration process. It can take up to 45-minutes to fully dissolve all of the initial CroFab vials (usually 4-6), so, start the process early (but after talking with poison control since it's really expensive stuff!)

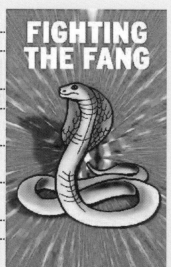

- Do not panic
- Reassure the victim
- Immobilise the affected limb with a cardboard splint and sticking tape
- Seek medical attention immediately
- Do not pick up the snake or try to trap it
- Do not apply a tight bandage around the wound
- Do not cut the wound with a knife/blade
- Do not suck out the venom
- Do not apply ice or immerse the wound in water

FIGHTING THE FANG

Don't: Ask the family to go back home and try to find or catch the snake so you can get a picture. In many cases, a brief verbal description is just fine, especially when paired with the geographic location, (e.g. Southwest Arizona vs. Alaska). But, do take a few minutes to learn about the most common venomous snakes in your area. Then, share that information and create a list to post somewhere in your ER.

Don't: Forget that there is no minimum age for CroFab. This means that if a baby is bit or a big person is bit, they get the same drug (and amazingly, the same dose as well). Because CroFab contains mercury, there may be some risk for a developing fetus. If given to a young child, there is a risk for neurological and renal toxicity; but, first and foremost, they must survive the bite! So in the ER, the antivenin CroFab can be administered across the lifespan.

Don't: Elevate the affected area. As the body part swells, one of the concerns is for compartment syndrome. And if blood is having a hard time going round and round because the tissues are getting squished, elevation just makes it <u>harder for blood</u> to go to that area. However, elevation makes it <u>easier for the toxin</u> to enter the blood stream and that's not a good thing. Immobilizing the limb – good! Elevating the limb – bad!

Don't: Apply a tourniquet. It doesn't help and can make perfusion to the extremity even worse. They are great for trauma - not for snake bites.

Don't: Suck out the poison. It's proven not to work and just sounds gross. No further explanation needed.

Just Remember

There are lots of Do's and Don'ts for snake bites. But the most important things are: 1) Call poison control first and 2) Be prepared if you hear someone saying, "Hold my beer and watch me catch this snake!"

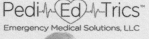

43

Peds Pearls

Something Doesn't Fit

DKA vs. Drugs

Scott DeBoer RN, MSN, CPEN, CEN, CFRN, CCRN, EMT-P
Founder of Pedi-Ed-Trics Emergency Medical Solutions, LLC

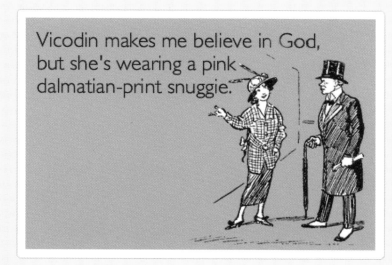

Vicodin makes me believe in God, but she's wearing a pink dalmatian-print snuggie.

It's inevitable… If you put a bunch of nurses or medics together at a wedding and give us a couple of margaritas, within three minutes we <u>will</u> start telling "war stories." So, here's one of my favorite and completely true, pediatric transport tales.

We were dispatched to transport a 2-year-old reported to be in new onset diabetic ketoacidosis (DKA). The patient was going from a community hospital ER to our pediatric ICU. The report that we received prepared us for an unconscious child with a Glasgow Coma Scale (GCS) of 5, intubated for respiratory depression, and hemodynamically stable. Her blood sugar was said to be 348, but of note, she had a blood gas with a normal pH and bicarb. After an unremarkable head CT, the community hospital staff was administering a normal saline bolus and beginning an insulin infusion. Our first thought was that something, *actually more than one thing*, doesn't fit!

Children in DKA rarely present acutely unconscious and very rarely have respiratory depression. Tachypnea and Kussmaul's... absolutely. Respiratory depression... not so much.

After landing, we (and in retrospect, the patient) were lucky enough to have the same paramedics who brought the child to the ER available and assigned to transport us from the helipad to the ER as well. In our brief discussions with them, they relayed that EMS had been called because of a child who had been found unresponsive that afternoon by the parents. The parents reported that the child had been well previously that morning. Even though our first thought was that everything is abuse until proven otherwise, there was no history or initial signs of trauma. The patient's blood sugar was >300 per finger stick in the ambulance, and she was unresponsive, "barely breathing," and had pinpoint pupils.

Does something stick out as "not right" about this scenario? The fact that she was fine that morning, was unresponsive a short while later, and had a normal pH and bicarb doesn't fit with DKA. Pinpoint pupils don't fit with DKA. Something, maybe too many things, don't fit…

Upon our assessment, the child had a GCS of 6 (without ER sedatives being given) and was not bucking the ventilator. Her skin was pink, warm and dry, and indeed she had pinpoint pupils. The parents denied being on any pain medications (specifically opiates such as Vicodin (hydrocodone), Dilaudid (hydromorphone), etc.), but they did mention that the grandmother who was babysitting the child that afternoon was being treated for chronic back pain. Bingo! One dose of Narcan (naloxone) later and the child sat up, tried to extubate herself, and the diagnosis was made. The child had gotten into Grandma's medications - OxyContin (oxycodone) as it turns out. Isn't it amazing how helpful a history can be!

An American Association of Poison Control Centers study found that 23% of prescribed medications ingested by kids under the age of five belonged to someone who didn't live in the household – and 17% of those belonged to a grandparent! A pediatric ER attending physician I love working with teaches that "Kids will ingest anything that doesn't eat them first … under and including the kitchen sink!"

The Moral of the Story… here is simple; If something doesn't fit, trust your gut. If you sense that something's not right, you are probably correct. It is our job to play detective (or call Dr. House) to figure out the solution to the puzzle.

VICODIN
Breakfast of Champions

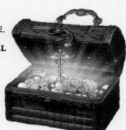

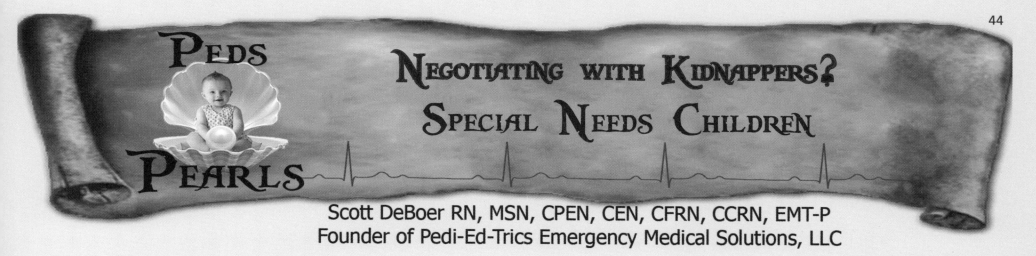

44

PEDS PEARLS

NEGOTIATING WITH KIDNAPPERS? SPECIAL NEEDS CHILDREN

Scott DeBoer RN, MSN, CPEN, CEN, CFRN, CCRN, EMT-P
Founder of Pedi-Ed-Trics Emergency Medical Solutions, LLC

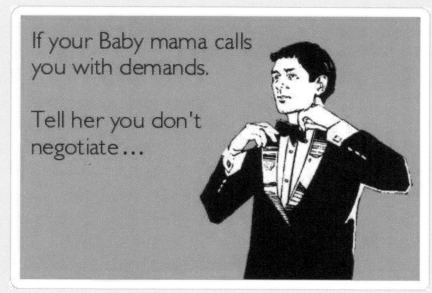

If your Baby mama calls you with demands.

Tell her you don't negotiate...

Doctor Mom (Or Dad...Or Caregiver...)

At a recent transport medicine conference, there was a truly great presentation on the EMS/ER management of special needs kids. Among the many valuable insights offered, one genuinely memorable gem from the presenter, Stu McVicar RRT, was brought forward by way of an unusual and thought-provoking question. That query was along the lines of, "What's the difference between a parent of a special needs child and a kidnapper?" The answer that was suggested was you can negotiate with a kidnapper! Indeed, you probably won't ever encounter a more steadfast, uncompromising, firm in their convictions individual than the parent of a special needs kid in an emergency situation. They've been there, done that, seen it all, and know what's best for their little ones. And you'd best believe them!

In the prehospital or ER worlds in which many of us live and play, a fair percentage of our "sick" kids are, honestly, not that sick. But, when you are dealing with a special needs kid who has chronic medical issues and gets sick, you take it up a notch. And that's a whole different story!

When caring for these special children and their very special parents, the tried and true approach is simply to ask Mom, Dad, or the primary caregiver if the situation has ever presented itself before. Chances are that your particular encounter is not the first. So, the logical follow-up question is to ask what was done the last time this happened. That's a great start. But don't stop there! Make sure to ask if it actually worked. No sense in repeating failures! And if you want bonus points, you can also ask the Mom (or Dad or caregiver), "What do you think we should do to fix this problem?" Ask the experts, the folks who play with, cope with, work with, care for, and pray for these special kids every day. Ninety-nine times out of a hundred, "Doctor Mom's" answer is exactly correct.

Think about children with autism: An individual with an autism disorder is commonly described as being on a spectrum (having a range of symptoms) or as having different levels of severity. At one of end is a severely affected child with developmental delays who is flapping and rocking. At the other end is a child with who can be described as being "a little quirky, but very bright." With one child, ritual and routine are everything. With the other, by simply asking what the child is interested in, you will be able to create a bond with the patient who, more than likely, will be happy to share with you an amazing amount of knowledge.

Think about children with shunts: It's very possible that the parents know more about this particular shunt than you do. They tend to know when something is wrong with the shunt and they certainly know when their kid is not acting normal or at least not at their baseline. Ask those all important questions and don't assume anything.

Think about children with tracheostomies and G-tubes: There is every chance the parents are very well versed about this particular trache or that specific G-tube. You may never have seen anything quite like it before or may never have seen that particular configuration, but it probably isn't new to the caregivers. They tend to know a great deal about these devices and know when something isn't quite right with the trache and/or G-tube. Believe the parents.

Think about children with "XYZ syndrome: "XYZ syndrome" may be something so new that you have never heard of it, or it might be something that the ED physician vaguely remembers reading about 20 years ago in medical school. Chances are that the parents in front of you are the regional experts on "XYZ syndrome" and in 60 seconds or less, they will teach you what you really need to know.

So... When it comes to special needs kids, simply ask Dr. Mom or Dr. Dad, and with time and patience, chances are you will be able to learn what you need to know and negotiating will be a thing of the past.

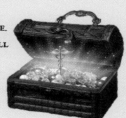

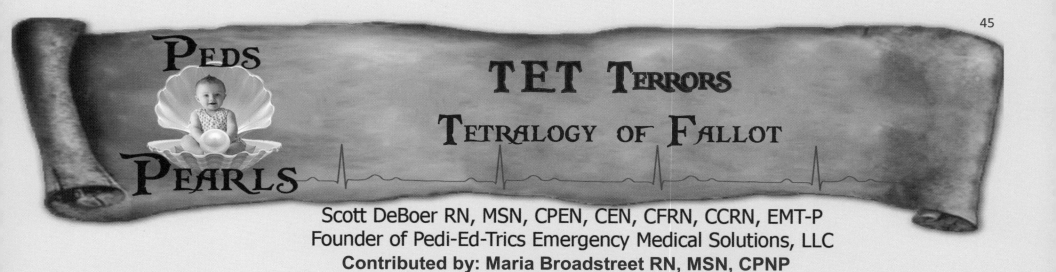

45

TET TERRORS
TETRALOGY OF FALLOT

Scott DeBoer RN, MSN, CPEN, CEN, CFRN, CCRN, EMT-P
Founder of Pedi-Ed-Trics Emergency Medical Solutions, LLC
Contributed by: Maria Broadstreet RN, MSN, CPNP

Blue Baby

From your position in the triage area, you can hear a screaming baby, who for some unknown reason, is not too happy to be in your ER (imagine that). He is crying at the top of his lungs as his mom runs over to you with her now "blue baby." Mom is understandably distraught and states, "He has tetralogy of Fallot. Please do something!!!" For those of you who have concerns over trying to make sense of congenital heart defects, don't fret. It's all about plumbing and where the blood flow is going. So, for a few moments, let's talk tetralogy.

Tetralogy (indicating four) of Fallot (doctor who named it) is a combination of four cardiac defects:

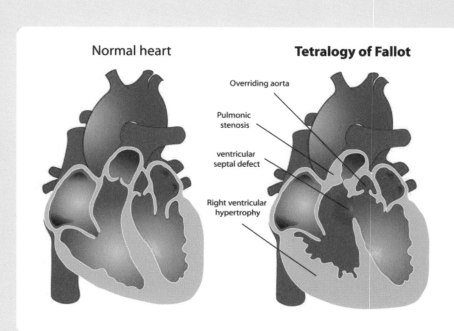

Normal heart

Tetralogy of Fallot

Overriding aorta

Pulmonic stenosis

ventricular septal defect

Right ventricular hypertrophy

1) **Pulmonary artery stenosis** (narrowing of the pulmonary artery)
   - The severity of this defect determines how sick your kid is going to be!!

2) **Ventricular septal defect** (hole between the ventricles)
   - This allows oxygenated (left side) and deoxygenated (right side) blood to mix resulting in overall lower blood oxygen saturations.

3) **Overriding aorta** (aorta straddles both the left and right ventricles)
   - This also allows oxygenated (left side) and deoxygenated (right side) blood to mix resulting in overall lower blood oxygen saturations.

4) **Right ventricular hypertrophy** (big right ventricle due to pumping against pulmonary stenosis)
   - This is a consequence of the right ventricle working way too hard.

These four defects mean that first, not enough blood is able to reach the lungs to get oxygen and second, poorly oxygenated blood flows out of the heart to the rest of the body. It may remain undiagnosed for days to weeks if the child has a persistently open big 'ol PDA (patent ductus arteriosus), aka the connection between aorta and pulmonary artery allowing blood to mix.

Pink and Blue

There are two types of tetralogy patients: "Pink TETs" and "Blue TETs."

1) **Pink TETs**: If you had to pick one, this is definitely the preferred kind of TET. These babies may have persistent mild desaturations (80-90%) or even normal oxygen saturations, hence, their coloring tends to be more "pink." The natural progression of a pink TET is to have slowly decreasing baseline oxygen saturations as they develop increasing right ventricular hypertrophy and narrowing around the pulmonary valve. These patients have a progressively harder time getting blood to the lungs so they start as a pink TET, but slowly evolve into a blue TET.

2) **Blue TETs**: These babies are cyanotic and stay cyanotic. They typically have severe pulmonary valve area stenosis (narrowing) or atresia (essentially, no valve). With the eventual closing of the PDA, they may turn blue and then stay blue as blood can no longer be shunted here, there, and everywhere. They usually need a cardiac surgical shunt/complete repair as soon as possible.

Either of these kinds of patients can have a TET spell during which they turn seriously blue. O_2 sats can drop to below 50%! This is a result of decreased blood flow to the lungs, most commonly from decreased systemic vascular resistance, and can be in response to agitation, crying, pooping, becoming dehydrated, or even just waking from a deep sleep.

To Be Continued...

Now that you understand the anatomy, in the next Peds Pearl, we will review the management of TET spells. On a side note, when you get home, grab some popcorn. There is a great movie called "*Something the Lord Made*" about the first cardiac surgical shunt operation for a one-year-old girl with tetralogy of Fallot. The year was 1944! It's kind of corny, but it provides a really great look at the history of pediatric cardiac surgery.

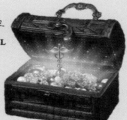

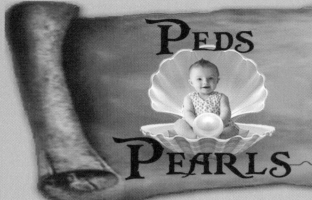

46

Stop, Drop, and Squat (or Sedate)
Tetralogy of Fallot and Tet Spells

Scott DeBoer RN, MSN, CPEN, CEN, CFRN, CCRN, EMT-P
Founder of Pedi-Ed-Trics Emergency Medical Solutions, LLC
Contributed by: Maria Broadstreet RN, MSN, CPNP

Blue Baby

From your position in the triage area, you can hear a screaming baby, who for some unknown reason, is not too happy to be in your ER (imagine that). He is crying at the top of his lungs as his mom runs over to you with her now "blue baby." Mom is understandably distraught and states, "He has tetralogy of Fallot. Please do something!!!"

Options...

You are now faced with this very blue and unstable infant in your triage area. What can you do to help this child and stop the spell?

- **Knee to Chest Position or Baby into a Ball**: Step 1 is to place the baby supine or chest-to-chest with an adult. Step 2, and this is the crucial one, is to bring the baby's knees up and tucked in close to the baby's chest. Bringing the legs up tight to the body may look like you've turned the baby into a ball and that's a good thing! If this can be done while the child is held snugly to the body of a familiar adult, it may have the added benefit of calming the child and helping to stop screaming. The key is that this positioning "kinks" off some of the blood flow to the lower half of the body, and thus, makes it easier for blood to go to the top half of the body, especially the lungs.

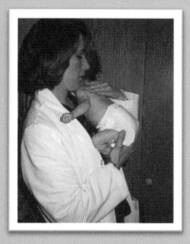

- **Squatting Position**: Older, undiagnosed TET children will often assume a squatting position to produce the same shunting to the lungs effect as the baby in a ball position. When something goes wrong and they are not getting enough blood to their lungs, they will "Stop, Drop, and Squat." Note: This is not seen much in the United States as most tetralogy of Fallot cases are diagnosed and repaired before the child's first birthday.

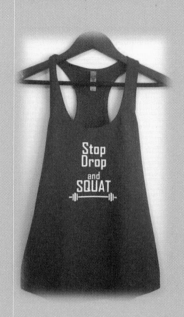

More Options....

Hopefully, squeezing or squatting will work, but, if not, here's some other EMS/ER options:

- **O₂**: The kid is purple. Feel free to give some oxygen. Even though the main issue is a physical obstruction to blood flow into the lungs, supplemental oxygen may have some benefit. Oxygen decreases pulmonary vascular resistance and hence, may help blood flow to the lungs if there is any open pathway to get there!

- **Sedation**: If you're thinking about IV sedation, hopefully your patient already has IV access because you DO NOT want to start an IV in a patient who is actively having a TET spell. That is simply because the more the child screams, the less blood gets to their lungs, and the more purple and clamped down they become. It's a vicious cycle and kids can die from a TET spell. If they have an IV, morphine is our drug of choice to mellow out a TET spell! Non-IV options include swaddling, sugar (TootSweet, Sweet-Ease, etc.), and intranasal medications such as Versed (midazolam) or Fentanyl.

- **Fluids**: If you already have an IV in place, consider giving the child a 10-20ml/kg fluid bolus. This helps increase the body's blood pressure and preload so more blood goes to the lungs. In addition, if you have given some IV sedation medications, the extra fluid may help ward off the evil "sedation induced hypotension" spirits. But, again, if you don't have IV access, this is not the time to rile up the kid with an invasive procedure if it can be avoided.

- **Prostaglandins (PGE₁)**: "Purple" begins with "P" and "Prostaglandins" also begin with "P." As detailed in another Peds Pearl about congenital heart disease, prostaglandins can help open a recently closed PDA or keep a PDA open if it is in the process of closing. This drug typically only works in the first week or so of life. But if you have a purple baby who is only a few days old and oxygen isn't making the baby less purple, the problem might be a funky heart and prostaglandins might be lifesaving!

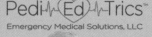

Info@PediEd.com 〰 1-888-280-PEDS (7337) 〰 PediEd.com

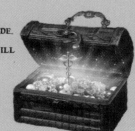

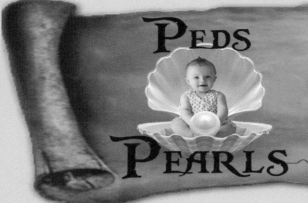

47

PEDS PEARLS

BEARING, BLOWING, AND BAGS

EMERGENCY MANAGEMENT OF PEDIATRIC SVT

Scott DeBoer RN, MSN, CPEN, CEN, CFRN, CCRN, EMT-P
Founder of Pedi-Ed-Trics Emergency Medical Solutions, LLC

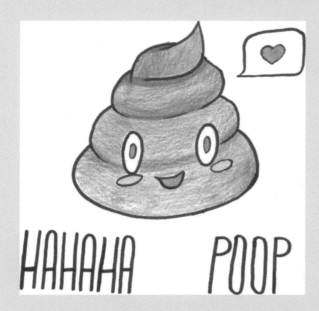

HAHAHA   POOP

Cute and Crashing

Pediatric patients **in supraventricular tachycardia** (SVT) come in two flavors – Cute or Crashing. The majority of kids in SVT are cute. They just happen to have a heart rate that's WAY too fast (over 220 beats per minutes for infants less than 1 year or over 180 for the rest of pediatric patients). If they are cute and able to express (verbally or otherwise) their lack of excitement about having paddles put on their chest for cardioversion, then they probably don't need to have paddles put on their chests. There are lots of other, non-electrical options available that work quite well in most kids.

Long before you give these cute SVT kids drugs which require IV access (and the mental gymnastics of calculating or locating the pediatric dose of adenosine), we urge you to consider some other things (hint: they are called vagal maneuvers) that you can try first. Hopefully, you would do this with your adult patients as well! And vagal maneuvers, like so many other things, come in two varieties, good ones and all the others.

Bad vagal maneuvers: Carotid massage or eyeball pressure. We all know that adults can have clogged up coronary arteries just waiting to cause heart attacks. Adults might also have clogged carotid arteries, just waiting to make the big time by sending clots downstream and causing a stroke. Carotid massage is a convenient way to dislodge some of those clots and doing anything that increases the likelihood of a stroke, most clinicians would agree, is just poor form. As far as the little ones who may not have the carotid clot problems (yet), just remember that these little ones have "Big head, little body (*and little or no palpable neck*) syndrome," so carotid massage just ain't gonna work. Eyeball massage just sounds wrong on many levels and as such, is no longer recommended. That was easy.

Good vagal maneuvers (young): Bearing. Telling adults to bear down (think childbirth, constipation, or the Chicago Bears theme song) can initiate a vagal response and temporarily drop their heart rate. But does asking kids to pretend that they are having a serious poop work particularly well? It might, if you can get them to stop laughing at you! So, consider the "bearing down" suggestion with older kids who are actually able to understand what you are asking them to do without breaking out in uncontrollable giggles and guffaws.

Good vagal maneuvers (younger): Blowing. Little kids tend to just laugh at you for saying "poop!" So, what works better in the little laughing kids (and older kids or adults as well)? Give them a drinking straw, crimp one end, and tell them to blow through the straw like there's no tomorrow. It achieves the same effect, but without having to potentially clean up the patient and the bed! Just a hint for you – Don't demonstrate the straw-blowing technique yourself unless you want to find yourself on the floor, or worse yet, on Facebook, as a result of a very effective vagal maneuver!

Good vagal maneuvers (youngest): Bags. So, in babies, we won't be doing carotid or eyeball massage. They bear down and poop all the time, just not on command. And straws are for chewing or sipping, not blowing. So, what works with babies in SVT? Evoke the mammalian diving reflex by placing a bag of crushed ice and/or ice water temporarily on the baby's forehead. You'll be needing a big response, so use a BIG bag, not just a small bag. It's important to remember to keep the nose and mouth open so the patient can still breathe. When you put the bag of ice suddenly on their forehead, it's like jumping into a really cold swimming pool. Gasping, followed by temporarily dropping their heart rate, are the anticipated responses. It's not pleasant by any means, but it works. So, if you really need that vagal thing, give it a try on those little ones. It's quick, easy, and only lasts a few seconds which is hopefully long enough to slow that speeding ticker!

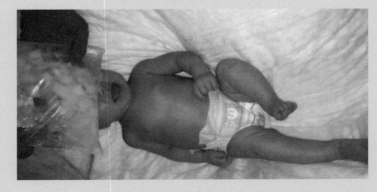

Your pearl for the kid with SVT is simple… Before you give them drugs or sedation followed by cardioversion, there's other things you can try first: **Bearing, Blowing, and Bags!**

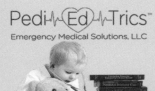

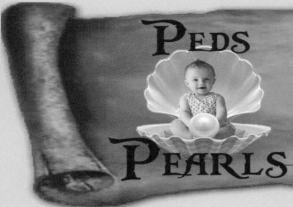

48

PEDS PEARLS

CALL 911 OR GO TO THE CLOSEST ER
TELEPHONE TRIAGE AND MEDICAL MALPRACTICE

Scott DeBoer RN, MSN, CPEN, CEN, CFRN, CCRN, EMT-P
Founder of Pedi-Ed-Trics Emergency Medical Solutions, LLC
Insights from: John Clark JD, MBA, NRP, FP-C, CCP-C, CMTE

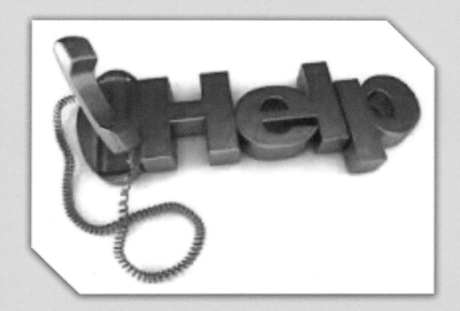

Red Flags

A recent medical-malpractice case involved a call to a pediatrician's office about an infant later diagnosed with meningitis. The infant was only a few weeks old and a key factor on the case was the way the phone call was handled. Simply put, you never want to see the words, "make an appointment" and "infant with fever" in the same telephone contact note. But that's indeed what happened and the story goes downhill from there.

The case plays out with a phone call to the pediatrician's office. Mom describes a three-week-old baby having a hard time breathing and a fever of 102°F (38.9°C). What are the big red flags here?

1) **3-week-old baby**

2) **Difficulty breathing**

3) **Fever!**

Essentially, the whole conversation, as was documented, is filled with big red flags saying something is not right: *Warning Will Robinson… Danger, Danger!*

So, if you're not sure what to suggest if a call like that comes in, let's start by saying that offering to make an appointment should <u>not</u> be one of those suggestions.

Appropriate phone advice:

In the ER, telephone advice is simple. Per recommendations from the American College of Emergency Physicians and the Emergency Nurses Association, *don't give it*. If the family member or patient feels there is a medical emergency, advise the person to call 911 or go to the nearest emergency department; anything else just sets the stage for something bad to happen.

As sometimes happens in the game of Monopoly, the message is "Do not pass go. Do not collect $200." Instead of going to jail, though, the caller seeking medical advice should go to the closest ER. There really is no second option.

Why is this the only option? Let's just say that when it comes to infants less than 28-days-old, nothing good ever comes of them having a fever. Once the infant arrives in the emergency department, here's what you can expect. The workup is simple - <u>everything</u>. That patient will get the whole septic workup including cathed urine for urinalysis and culture, CBC and a blood culture, chest X-ray, and the dreaded lumbar puncture. Why? Because when babies are transitioning from "life is good inside of Mom" to the harsh outside world, the chance of catching something icky that might kill them is pretty good until their immune system is up to snuff. So, during the first month of life, every baby with a documented rectal temp greater than or equal to 100.4°F (38.0°C) is septic until proven otherwise. And if they're not septic, it's because they are thinking about becoming septic.

In many ER's, infants under 28-days of age are triaged as level II, or even level I! This means that it's "all hands on deck" as the baby gets assessed, cultured, and administered antibiotics ASAP. Recommendations across the board are that neonatal patients presenting with these symptoms are a hospital admission until we figure out what is going on.

So, any communication regarding a 3-week-old with a fever (and hence, possibly septic) that suggests anything except the need for an immediate trip to the ER, just implies to Mom that this is not a time critical issue and sets the stage for a potentially really bad outcome.

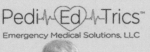

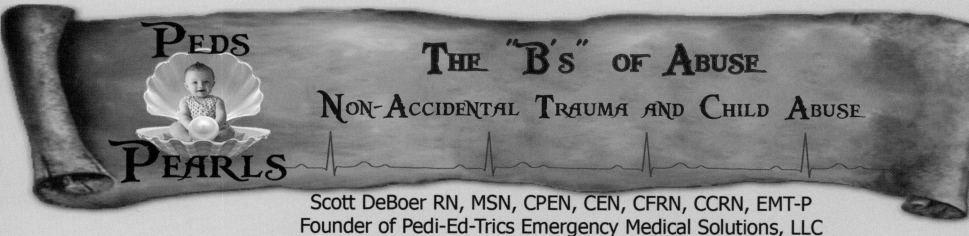

The "B's" of Abuse
Non-Accidental Trauma and Child Abuse

Scott DeBoer RN, MSN, CPEN, CEN, CFRN, CCRN, EMT-P
Founder of Pedi-Ed-Trics Emergency Medical Solutions, LLC

Six "B's" Of Abuse

Years ago, a brilliant pediatric trauma coordinator from a children's hospital in Chicago taught me what she called her "Six B's of Abuse." They are – Bumps, Bruises, Breaks, Burns, Bites, and Bathrooms.

Bumps – While it may seem self-explanatory, bear in mind that some bumps are to be expected with little ones. But bumps in unusual places or areas where it seems hard to be bumped, should be considered suspicious.

Bruises – Bumps can lead to bruises and this is not entirely unexpected. But consider all the factors and available information. If the history doesn't fit, or if different stages of healing are present, is there a pattern that emerges? And what does that pattern suggest?

Breaks – Many of us survived childhood without any broken bones. But if broken bones in kids were really rare, we wouldn't see all those cool colors and patterns of casting material. But again, consider the story, the history, and even some of the subtle factors presented by the child and guardian. And certainly, breaks in children who have limited mobility are inherently suspicious.

Burns– The history and presentation of burns provide many needed clues as to the level of suspicion that we attribute to them. Consider the size and mobility of the child involved. Does the story make sense? Is it even possible, let alone plausible? Does the actual presentation fit the history? Are there unusual splash patterns? Are there burn marks in areas that should have been protected by clothing? Are there multiple signs of burns in different stages of healing? Is there a visible pattern that emerges?

Bites – It should go without saying that human bite marks (especially adult size bite marks) in any location are worthy of being reported. Other sorts of bites may also be indicative of abuse, though it may be animal instead of human abuse.

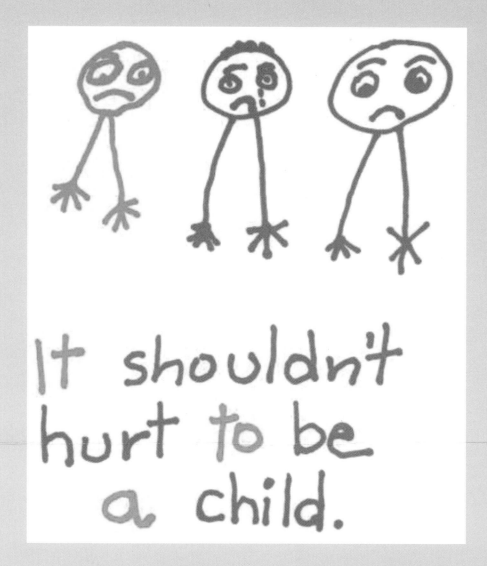

It shouldn't hurt to be a child.

The first five B's instinctively make sense, but the **Bathroom**? When you look at parents who snap and abuse their kids, one of the big instigators is all the stressors associated with toilet training. So, complaints related to bathroom activities, such as painful urination, painful defecation, or constipation may have origins in abusive situations.

For years, she taught her "Six B's of Abuse," and recently, she has added one more - the "**Bikini** bathing suit." Children who have an injury somewhere that should be specifically covered by the equivalent of a girl's bikini or a boy's swimsuit should raise a big red flag for possible abuse.

The B's of Abuse: Bumps, Bruises, Breaks, Burns, Bites, Bathrooms, and Bikinis

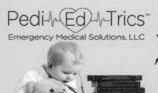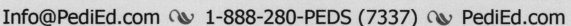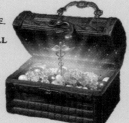

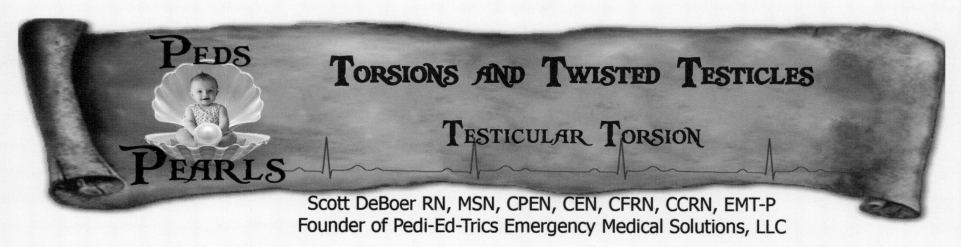

50

PEDS PEARLS

TORSIONS AND TWISTED TESTICLES

TESTICULAR TORSION

Scott DeBoer RN, MSN, CPEN, CEN, CFRN, CCRN, EMT-P
Founder of Pedi-Ed-Trics Emergency Medical Solutions, LLC

Scenario:

A recent pediatric case involved a 12-year-old child who required emergency surgery at 2 a.m. Before he went to the OR, the urology attending physician gave the Emergency Department staff a brilliant, 30-second in-service which we considered to be his response to the question: "*Under what conditions should you wake me up at 2 a.m.?*"

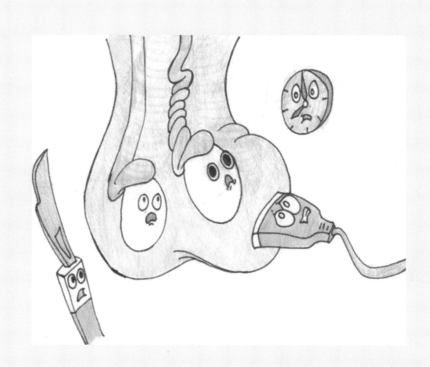

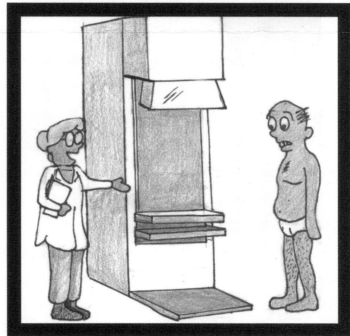

"*Okay, [Jim]. Just stick it in between those two devices.*"

If Women Ran the World

Twisted Testicles

His take on twisted testicles was totally simple, very easy to remember… and it really works. It is a true medical emergency when:

1) You have a 12-year-old boy who actually admits to having a problem "down there." The reasoning is simple. If you are a teenage boy, the last thing in the world you EVER want to discuss, or even worse, seek medical care for, is a problem "down there."

2) The pain is so bad that they barf. That part is self-explanatory.

Time is Tissue

Many urologists still prefer to have confirmation of torsion made via ultrasound before waking up, coming in, and going to surgery. But if the patient is male and hurts so bad that he vomits (combined with the location of the pain being "down there"), your patient probably has a torsion. Get a stat ultrasound and give a heads up to urology and the OR right away. Time is muscle for MI's. Time is brain for strokes. And time is tissue for testicles!

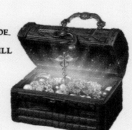

Info@PediEd.com ✆ 1-888-280-PEDS (7337) ✆ PediEd.com

51

PEDS PEARLS

VOLVULUS BEGINS WITH V

ASSESSMENT AND MANAGEMENT OF PEDIATRIC VOLVULUS

Scott DeBoer RN, MSN, CPEN, CEN, CFRN, CCRN, EMT-P
Founder of Pedi-Ed-Trics Emergency Medical Solutions, LLC

V is for Very Bad

Volvulus begins with "V" and it's very, very bad! It is caused by the intestine partially or completely twisting around itself and can quickly result in intestinal ischemia, necrosis, peritonitis, perforation, and even death!

Several years ago, I served as an expert witness on a medical-malpractice case involving an infant who was no more than a few days old. The infant, according to the documentation, presented with a suspected volvulus. That simple phrase was a key factor in the case. Essentially, a significant consideration in the case was that you never want to see the words "waiting room" and "suspected volvulus" in the same sentence (or even together anywhere on the chart!)

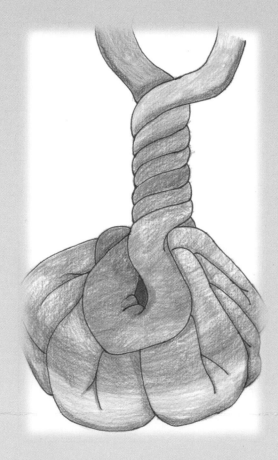

Volvulus is most commonly a result of a **congenital intestinal malrotation** and when it occurs, it is typically found in children less than one-year of age. It is most definitely a life-threatening condition and <u>must</u> be triaged that way. What we look for is the infant who arrives because Mom says that the baby is not eating well and has been spitting up lots of "green stuff." Remember, if you are feeding a very, very young one, there probably isn't anything "green" in the diet. Therefore, nothing "green" should be coming back out from above. That is a crucial point. Green out of any baby's orifices is not normal and <u>nothing</u> good comes of a little one spitting up green. So, first the baby spits up lots of icky green stuff (referred to as forceful bilious vomiting), then their belly looks icky (referred to as distended, tense, with hypoactive or absent bowel sounds), then the whole baby looks icky (referred to as very, very sick). Unfortunately, when babies look that icky, for whatever reason, death may be waiting just around the corner. So, the waiting room is clearly <u>not</u> where they belong.

So, clinically speaking, symptoms leading to the suspicion of volvulus in an infant should include:

1) Bilious vomiting

2) Acute and constant abdominal pain

3) Lots of air in the proximal small intestine coupled with abdominal distension

4) A really sick (i.e., trying to die) and shocky general appearance.

The life-threatening progression of this condition is actually quite simple. Volvulus is a twisted portion of the gut that can lead to an ischemic portion of gut. Ischemic gut can quickly lead to dead gut. Dead gut can quickly lead to a dead baby!

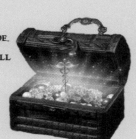
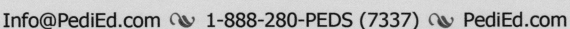

52

PEDS PEARLS

WHAT SIZE, HOW MUCH, AND WHERE... EVERY KID, EVERY TIME
AIRWAYS, EPINEPHRINE, AND INTRAOSSEOUS

Scott DeBoer RN, MSN, CPEN, CEN, CFRN, CCRN, EMT-P
Founder of Pedi-Ed-Trics Emergency Medical Solutions, LLC
Insights from: Joie Hickenbottom RN, EMT-P, CEN

Expect the Unexpected

When our transport team is orienting new residents or working with new nurses, we emphasize the need to expect the unexpected. As a key part of that thinking, we strongly recommend the "What size, how much, and where" rule for every kid, every time. Whether the kid is sick or not sick, big or little, pink or purple... Always ask, "What size, how much, and where."

- **What size**: With every kid, s/he may look cute now, but if they crash 2 minutes later, what size endotracheal tube are you going to place?

- **How much**: With every kid, s/he may look cute now, but if they crash 2 minutes later, how much epi are you going to push?

- **Where**: With every kid, s/he may look cute now, but if they crash 2 minutes later, where are you going to place the IO (intraosseous needle)?

Intraosseous Devices

Years ago, placing an intraosseous device was pretty much limited to skills labs (where many chicken legs were sacrificed in the name of education) or, heaven forbid, attempts to resuscitate a baby at the brink of death. But that was then, and this is now. These days we teach, preach, and perform the skill of placing IOs on patients of all ages from babes in the cradle to senior citizens.

In our experience, the most common reason people don't like placing IO devices is because our colleagues aren't confident about finding the correct landmarks. You can start by palpating the following insertion landmarks on both legs and both arms:

- Proximal humerus (especially in kids over 10-years old)
- Distal femur (peds only)
- Proximal and Distal tibia on EVERYONE

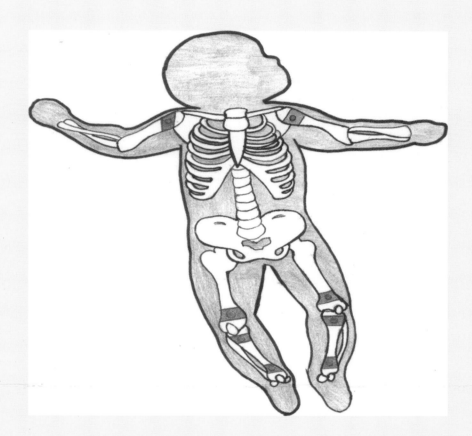

You are going to have to do a physical exam on them anyway, so when you are doing your exam, simply feel their arms and legs and find the spots.

Plan Ahead

In the ED or ICU, on EVERY patient, whether a hangnail vs. a multi-system trauma patient, it's a good idea to plan ahead… to expect the unexpected. If you figure out these three things: tube sizes, drug doses, and found landmarks with <u>every</u> kid, <u>every</u> time, by the time a child unexpectedly crashes, you will have prepared *hundreds*, if not *thousands* of times. It will be second nature for you and your colleagues! Your first 999 patients won't need it, but patient 1,000 will be glad you were able to quickly calculate what size, how much, and where!

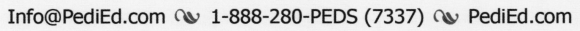

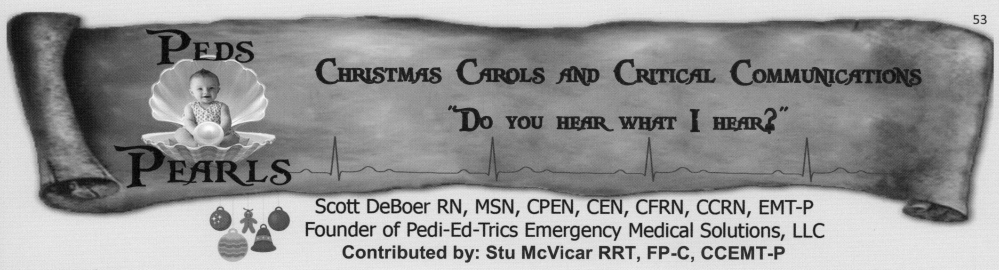

53

Christmas Carols and Critical Communications
"Do you hear what I hear?"

Scott DeBoer RN, MSN, CPEN, CEN, CFRN, CCRN, EMT-P
Founder of Pedi-Ed-Trics Emergency Medical Solutions, LLC
Contributed by: Stu McVicar RRT, FP-C, CCEMT-P

During the Christmas season, it's a virtual certainty that you will hear the refrain, "… do you see what I see… do you hear what I hear?" Interestingly, these words from a popular Christmas carol work equally well as a reminder about communicating crucial elements of pediatric assessments.

All too often, when a call goes out for an emergency pediatric transport, whether by ground or by air, one of the challenges faced by the on-call team is getting the most useful report concerning the condition of the patient. Over the radio or telephone, the on-scene EMS or ED professionals might relay information like "the respiratory rate is 28 and the sats are 94%..." A short time later, when the transport team arrives and first sees the patient in person, they are presented with a child, quite obviously in severe respiratory distress, and who REALLY is WORKING to achieve that sat of 94%. Suprasternal, intercostal, supraclavicular, and subcostal retractions are all present despite albuterol treatments and subcutaneous epinephrine. The assessment of lung sounds reveals next to nothing and that's scary bad. A "silent chest" with little to no audible air movement is an ominous sign. Scariest of all is the fact that the young child does not fight having an oxygen mask strapped to his face and only has a weak cry in response to his finger stick blood sugar test!

After transports, teams often call (or get calls from) the sending group to provide an update on how the flight went and how the child was doing in the Pediatric ICU. In cases like those mentioned above, it's hard not to ask why nothing was mentioned about the obvious retractions, silent chest, and sleepy status. Sometimes, even without prompting, the transport team learns that the senders knew that things really were looking scary, but they didn't want to sound like things weren't under control or they didn't want to sound stupid broadcasting improper medical terminology.

If you can't remember the fancy medical terms, that's OK. Just tell the transport team what you are seeing and hearing. Being on the receiving end, which of the following reports would you want to get?

1) Our patient has a RR of 28 and a sat of 94%.

2) I can count every one of his ribs when he takes a breath in. You could eat soup out of his breast bone; it's getting sucked in so deep! His nostrils look like an angry pig when he's working to breathe! And oh yeah, he ain't moving squat for air and is seriously sleepy!

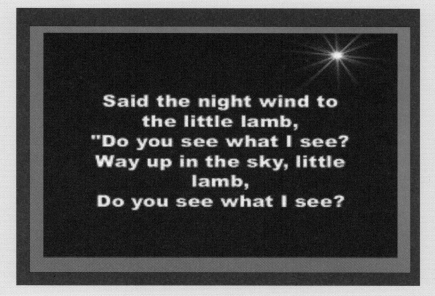

Said the night wind to the little lamb, "Do you see what I see? Way up in the sky, little lamb, Do you see what I see?

In the first example, the focus is on the numbers. And depending on the age of the child, those numbers may be perfectly normal. Though not a single medical term is used in the second example, there is no doubt about what's going on with the patient. It paints a picture of a child in SEVERE respiratory distress and impending respiratory failure - a child who is slipping away from the land of the living.

The first three verses of that Christmas carol should guide your report. Do you see what I see… do you hear what I hear… do you know what I know? Tell the transport team (and anyone else caring for this patient) what you are seeing, hearing (or not hearing), and what you know. Don't worry about fancy medical terminology. Saying that "the kid looks sick as a dog, needs an airway, and is about to code" will certainly get any transport team's attention and does a great job of telling them what you hear and what you see!

An extra note from Scott:

If possible, please relay the approximate age of the kid, the approximate weight, or even better, both. As everything in kids is based on age and/or weight (in kilos), it really makes the transport team's job much easier if they have a rough guestimate as to age and/or weight before arriving.

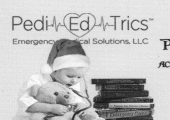

Info@PediEd.com ✆ 1-888-280-PEDS (7337) ✆ PediEd.com